Fresh & Fermented

85 Delicious Ways to Make Fermented Carrots, Kraut, and Kimchi Part of Every Meal

JULIE O'BRIEN & RICHARD J. CLIMENHAGE
Photography by Charity Burggraaf

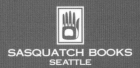

SASQUATCH BOOKS
SEATTLE

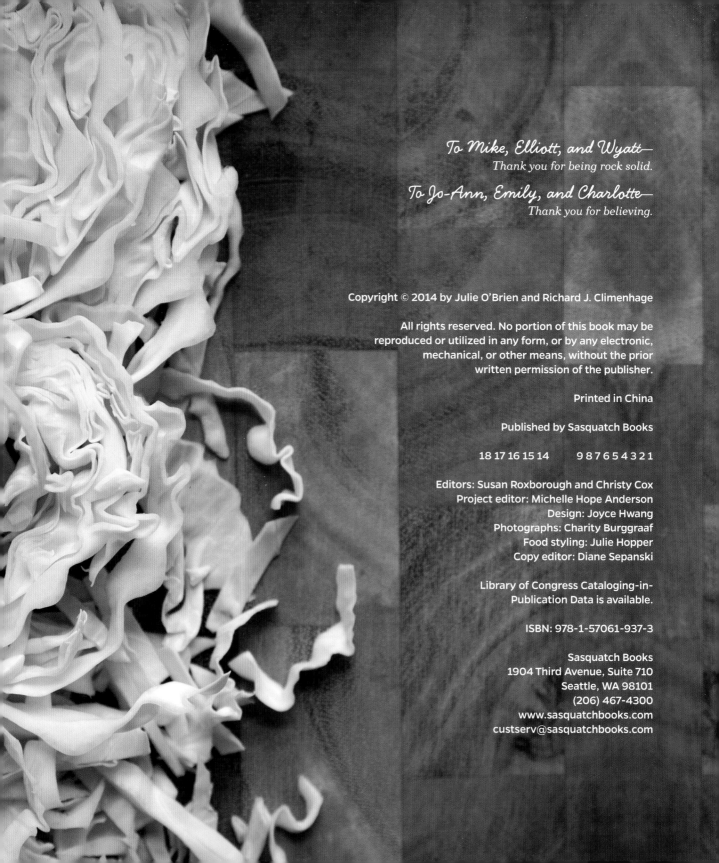

To Mike, Elliott, and Wyatt—
Thank you for being rock solid.

To Jo-Ann, Emily, and Charlotte—
Thank you for believing.

Printed in China

Published by Sasquatch Books

18 17 16 15 14   9 8 7 6 5 4 3 2 1

Editors: Susan Roxborough and Christy Cox
Project editor: Michelle Hope Anderson
Design: Joyce Hwang
Photographs: Charity Burggraaf
Food styling: Julie Hopper
Copy editor: Diane Sepanski

Library of Congress Cataloging-in-Publication Data is available.

ISBN: 978-1-57061-937-3

Sasquatch Books
1904 Third Avenue, Suite 710
Seattle, WA 98101
(206) 467-4300
www.sasquatchbooks.com
custserv@sasquatchbooks.com

Contents

Recipe List

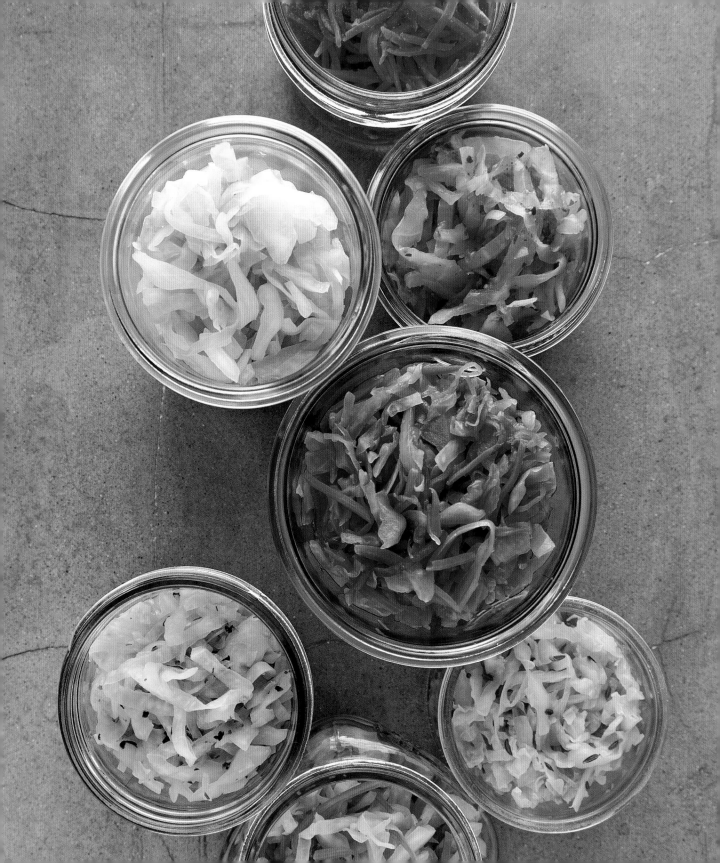

Introduction

What if there was a food you could eat every day, in every meal, that would amaze you with its flavor while it nurtured and healed your body? What if this food were inexpensive and simple to make? And what if it were also essential to healthy digestion, helping you get the most out of the nutrients in the foods you eat?

This wondrous food exists! It's good old-fashioned, raw-fermented vegetables. Celebrated by cultures around the world and integral to cuisines for thousands of years, this age-old food-preserving technique is reclaiming its rightful place in kitchens today.

In *Fresh & Fermented*, we'll teach you how to make your own small-batch fermented veggies with the award-winning flavors of the products from Firefly Kitchens. You don't need much to get going—a few very basic tools, some fresh vegetables, pure sea salt, and spices. We'll give you detailed instructions and tips based on our broad experience to set you confidently on your way. By planning ahead and letting Mother Nature do the work, you can have a jar of tangy, fresh ferments on your counter at all times.

After you've made your first jar of kraut, you'll find more than eighty mouth watering ways you can put it to good use. Our home-tested recipes are written with an attention to detail that can help even the most novice cook turn out delicious meals. Transform your breakfasts; add zip to dips, salads, and sandwiches;

and boost the vitality of dinners and sparkle of desserts. And the recipes don't stop there—they'll inspire you with ideas for how you can adapt everyday foods to incorporate fermented veggies and give you plenty of permission to experiment. We like a tablespoon or three of kraut at every meal. These recipes allow you to incorporate those servings in ways you'd never imagine.

In these pages, you'll also learn a bit of the science behind fermentation—about the bacteria that make it happen, the critical and integral role they play in our digestion and immune systems, and the incredible health benefits and healing powers that these beneficial bacteria (called *probiotics*) confer.

We *live* kraut every single day—we make it, jar it, sell it, talk about it, and teach people to make it. The more we listened to the stories of our customers and friends across the country about how kraut has changed their lives, the more we realized just how little was known about this incredibly healthy food, and how few people were eating it. How could we keep this delicious and healthful secret to ourselves? We wanted both to tell people about it and empower them to *do* something about it.

So we wrote *Fresh & Fermented* to bring the bright magic of fermented foods from Firefly Kitchens into your kitchen at home.

—JULIE O'BRIEN & RICHARD CLIMENHAGE

The Story of Firefly Kitchens

In January 2011, in San Francisco's historic Ferry Building, we—Julie and Richard— proudly accepted a Good Food Award for one of our most popular products, Yin Yang Carrots. We were glowing with delight at being honored by an award that celebrates tasty, authentic, handcrafted foods—products that are responsibly produced and build strong local communities. Alice Waters, a famed proponent of these values, spoke at the awards ceremony. She talked specifically about traditional foods and how far we as a nation have strayed from making them. Only one year into business, we were thrilled to be recognized as outstanding in a field of a hundred other like-minded producers.

Four years later we're reflecting on that experience, and the successive Good Food Awards our products have received. Although we've had to work harder than we ever imagined, we are still amazed by what we have accomplished with just a few ambitious ideas and in so little time. Now, with more than one hundred thousand jars of kraut, kimchi, and other fermented veggies behind us, multiple awards for our repertoire, and opportunities to share some of our knowledge, we are feeling immensely grateful for our ability to do and share what we love. That is what *Fresh & Fermented* is all about.

We started Firefly Kitchens in 2010 to bring our collective knowledge and passion together to create a line of naturally fermented products. For almost a year we used regular kitchen tools, rental kitchen space, and ceramic crocks to ferment small batches of kraut that we sold at local farmers' markets. After that start-up year, we moved into our own commercial kitchen space, with fermentation tanks many times the size of our former crocks.

Backing and support from Whole Foods Market's Local Producer Loan Program allowed us to take the next steps toward growth and expansion, and we spent 2012 scaling up our production to meet the new and growing needs of local and regional stores. By the end of 2013, we had successfully quadrupled our sales and distribution. As we bring 2014 to a close, we're sending our products off to retail locations throughout Washington, Oregon, California, Nevada, Arizona, Hawaii, and western Canada.

We've fermented over sixty tons of organic and sustainably grown vegetables, sourced primarily from local, family-owned organic farms. We've stuck to our small-batch principle, keeping the quality of all our products the best we possibly can.

Our experience at Firefly Kitchens has enabled us to teach hundreds of people how to make their own fermented foods. We've given talks and shared recipes with students of health and nutrition, opening the eyes of the next generation to age-old fermentation traditions. We've hosted team-building meetings for companies who send their employees to our kitchen for a day to share new experiences (packing jars and affixing labels), learn about the fermentation process, taste new flavors—and build more cohesive teams in the process. We've regularly celebrated with community members at our fermented happy hours, which have evolved from a small gathering of friends to a collaboration between Firefly and other local producers to share an amazing spread of food, drinks, and other goods.

Throughout it all, our kitchen has remained open to anyone and everyone interested in helping, learning, and sharing with us, and it's this support from our community that has helped us thrive. From long days of stuffing hundreds of jars with fermented veggies to short visits from friends sharing their favorite new way to eat Firefly's ferments, our passion for microbe-rich foods and the support and enthusiasm of our community of volunteers and friends have pushed us onward.

Even people who claim they dislike sauerkraut love our ferments—"They taste so *fresh*!" But the most rewarding aspect of our work is the countless stories that come from so many people who tell us they "just feel better" from eating our fermented cabbage and carrots. We regularly get calls from people who explain that their long-standing digestive discomfort has disappeared after they started eating just a small amount of fermented foods each day. People with compromised immune function tell us they find remedy in our nutrient-dense products, joining the many others who, for many reasons, look to fermented foods to improve their health.

Fresh & Fermented is just part of our response to continued requests for more products in more places and in more forms. Whether for health, taste, or both, we want to show you how you can eat better, feel better, and live better no matter where you are. All of us at Firefly Kitchens hope that what you eat will make you glow!

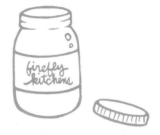

Chapter 1:
Fermentation, Good Bacteria & Good Health

FROM THE DAWN OF RECORDED HISTORY, humans have been fermenting foods—meat, milk, wheat, fruits, and vegetables. Many, perhaps all, civilizations have harnessed fermentation to reliably and safely preserve foods. Archaeological evidence suggests that the earliest ferments were alcoholic beverages: Neolithic peoples in China made alcoholic beverages from rice, fruit, and honey, and ceramic vases from around 5000 BC found in modern-day Iran show traces of wine.

A fermented food is one whose taste and texture have been transformed by the introduction of beneficial bacteria or yeast. If you've eaten yogurt, salami, cheese, chocolate, or kimchi, or drunk coffee, wine, whiskey, or beer, you've enjoyed the edible pleasures of fermentation.

Of course, fermented foods taste great—vibrant, with heady aromas, extraordinary flavors, and appealing textures—but they also play an important role in our bodies. Fermentation partially breaks down food, making the nutrients easier for our bodies to assimilate and the vitamins, enzymes, and minerals more available for us to digest. Fermented foods supply vitamin C and help produce essential vitamins that our bodies cannot make, such as vitamin K and B-complex vitamins. Fermentation also defends our digestive system against harmful bacteria by creating an environment that's too acidic for their survival.

Bacteria in Fermentation

Fermentation is initiated in one of two ways: either by introducing yeast or bacteria into the food to be fermented through a starter culture (such as whey) or naturally, by microorganisms in the environment or already on the food (the Firefly Kitchens approach).

CAN PEOPLE WHO ARE LACTOSE INTOLERANT EAT FOODS THAT RESULT FROM LACTO-FERMENTATION?

Lacto-fermentation takes its name from lactic acid bacteria that produce *lactic acid* as a by-product of digesting the sugar in vegetables. Don't confuse it with *lactose*, which is found in milk. Any vegetables fermented with salt won't give you digestive problems resulting from lactose intolerance.

Bacteria convert starches, sugars, and other nutrients into alcohols or acids—one of those being lactic acid. Fermentation that produces lactic acid is called lactic acid fermentation (or *lacto-fermentation*). The main player in lactic acid fermentation is a group of bacteria called lactic acid bacteria (or *lactobacilli*). They're present on the surface of living things—in fact, almost all vegetables are naturally endowed with a plentiful supply of these bacteria. Lactic acid bacteria are not the only bacteria that can create fermentation; they're just the ones most commonly found on cabbage and the other vegetables that we ferment at Firefly Kitchens and that are the subject of this book.

Bacteria in Our Bodies

The lactic acid bacteria that ferment food are also present in, and interact with, the bacteria in our bodies.

Our bodies are alive with bacteria, bacteria that have been with us from the moment we were born. For every cell in our bodies, there are ten indigenous bacteria: the body is made up of about 10 trillion cells, but the bacteria there number more than 100 trillion. Our bodies are hosts to hundreds of species of these bacteria, giving them a home, an environment in which to thrive. At the same time we are completely dependent on bacteria to sustain essential processes, in particular those of the digestive and immune systems. We are, in effect, codependent species.

Bacteria are found outside and inside our bodies, but 80 percent of them (by some estimates, two to three *pounds*) live in the gastrointestinal tract, particularly the large intestine.

Bacteria and the digestive system

A properly functioning digestive system is the bedrock of good health. The digestive system extracts nutrients from the food we eat by breaking it down, both mechanically and chemically, ultimately reducing food to its essential nutrients—molecules small enough to be absorbed by our cells to nourish our bodies. We nourish ourselves, then, not so much by what we eat, but by what our bodies can absorb and use as nutrients. The best diet in the world won't help if our bodies can't digest what we eat.

So how does digestion work? The digestive system is a complex ecosystem that involves interplay between the organs (such as the stomach and intestines) and bacteria in our bodies.

When we take the first bite, the teeth and tongue mechanically break down the food while taste and smell trigger salivary glands to produce enzymes that start the digestion of starches. When we swallow, the partially digested food goes into the stomach, where highly acidic gastric juices further break down the food, the main function of the stomach.

Lactic acid bacteria help regulate the acidity of the stomach, stimulating production when levels drop, and suppressing production when they're elevated. Lactic acid bacteria also produce acetylcholine, which stimulates the stomach's digestive muscles to push the food into the intestines (or gut). The gut is where our bodies absorb most of the food's nutrients, including vitamins and minerals.

There are hundreds of species of bacteria in the gut, including lactic acid bacteria, which are vital to good digestion. It's bacteria that break down complex carbohydrates into digestible sugars and starches. Bacteria synthesize vitamins such as vitamin A, B-complex vitamins, and vitamin K, and secrete compounds that may help in the absorption of essential minerals such as calcium, magnesium, and iron. Without this bacterial activity, these nutrients would go undigested—and unused. Bacteria also break down fiber (which we cannot digest) and use it to fuel their own growth.

Bacteria and the immune system

Beyond the influence of bacteria in nutrition, a substantive body of research points to the critical and integral role that intestinal bacteria play in the immune system, the bulk of which resides in the gut. Recent studies have shown that the state of our gut bacteria has a profound effect on the active states of the immune cells in our intestinal lining.

There are two parts to the immune system. The protective component (the innate immune system) is a physical barrier that prevents pathogens and other harmful elements from entering the body. The responsive component (the selective immune system) goes into action when the protective defenses fail. The lining of the digestive tract plays a role in both parts.

In its protective role, the digestive tract lining works like the walls guarding a medieval city. The defensive power of the walls depends on how many gates and other openings there are (its permeability), and how many sentinels the city has to defend those openings (the immune response). Studies have shown that having a healthy array of gut bacteria can reduce intestinal permeability (the number of gates) and increase immune cell function (the guards) in the gut lining.

The lining of the digestive tract also plays a responsive role in the immune system. Recent studies show that the makeup of the bacterial community in the gut can activate the immune cells in the intestinal walls. Researchers in Japan, for example, recently discovered that *Clostridium* bacteria release an acid that activates white blood cells in the lining of the intestine, alerting the body to prepare its defenses against pathogens.

The bacterial community in our bodies is essential to life. However, the research into the fundamental part that bacteria play is relatively recent, and we live in a society that has taught us to believe that bacteria are uniformly "bad," and that has waged a decades-long war to eliminate them.

The Dark Side of Germ Phobia

Daily, we hear messages from the medical profession, government agencies such as the U.S. Food and Drug Administration (FDA), pharmaceutical companies, and food manufacturers warning us about the dangers of bacteria. We listen to ads for antibacterial room fresheners, mouthwashes, and household cleaning products that promise to destroy bacteria (99.9 percent!).

Antibiotics are pervasive. Our children take courses of antibiotics to clear up ear infections or acne. If we eat meat or drink cow's milk, we may consume antibiotics because they're mixed into the food of commercially bred animals. Fruits and vegetables may absorb antibiotics if they're fertilized with manure from cows fed antibiotics. Antibiotics are even found in our water supply.

Of course, antibiotics (and other germicidal measures) were developed to protect us from harmful bacteria, and they have saved the lives of millions. But there is a dark side to the story. Antibiotics are often indiscriminate, destroying not only pathogens, but beneficial bacteria in our bodies as well. Research has also shown that the use of antibiotics can cause bacteria to mutate so they become resistant to antibiotics. Some antibiotics lead to the growth of yeasts (like *Candida albicans*) that suppress the immune system.

Anything that destroys bacteria can compromise the ability of the beneficial bacteria in our bodies to help us absorb the food we eat, and can throw off the balance of our immune systems. Without a lively environment of beneficial bacteria, harmful species can proliferate, further weakening the body.

EATING FERMENTED FOODS CAN IMPROVE DIGESTION

"I have suffered from poor digestion my whole life, and several autoimmune diseases had wiped out my gut to an extreme. When I began eating Firefly raw kraut, I noticed an immediate difference. If I go several days without kraut, my system is not happy!"

—BETSY POWER

"I have always had a sensitive stomach—kind of a drag as a chef. No disease or condition, just touchy. From the first time I tried the naturally fermented Firefly krauts, I noticed a relaxing feeling in my gut. Like a fist unclenching. Like my stomach was going *ahhhhhh!* This soothed and eased feeling has made me an ardent fan. I try to eat Firefly krauts several times a day and always drink all of the brine, as well."

—NICOLE ALONI

Fermented foods can temper the negative effects of these stresses on our native bacterial community, blunting the attack on our bacteria and bolstering our defenses against disease.

The Benefits of Lacto-Fermented Foods

People have long believed in the health advantages of eating fermented foods. For example, it's thought that Tiberius, one of Rome's greatest generals and emperor from AD 14 to 37, traveled with salted cabbage to protect his soldiers from disease. The American Civil War physician John Jay Terrell, who treated prisoners of war, credited his success in lowering his patients' death rate to the raw sauerkraut that he added to their diets. Dr. Élie Metchnikoff, a Russian biologist who won the Nobel Prize in 1908 for his pioneering research on the immune system, identified the potential of lactic acid bacteria to lengthen life.

Today, research shows that lacto-fermented foods alive with lactic acid bacteria bestow many health benefits on us. You'll hear these bacteria referred to as *probiotics*, microbes that benefit us when we eat them. Probiotics predigest nutrients, manufacture and supply us with vitamins, and may be used to cure specific illnesses.

PROBIOTICS PREDIGEST NUTRIENTS. Lactic acid bacteria in fermented foods, as a result of their own digestive activity, break down the carbohydrates and other nutrients we eat into simpler components. The bacteria work like biological food processors, breaking down the cell walls of our food so the body doesn't have to work as hard to digest it. This is particularly beneficial to those with impaired digestive systems or those who suffer from digestive problems.

PROBIOTICS MANUFACTURE AND SUPPLY US WITH VITAMINS. Lactic acid bacteria, one kind of probiotics, manufacture the full complex of B vitamins, including thiamin (B_1), riboflavin (B_2), and niacin (B_3). B-complex vitamins are essential to the body for many reasons, such as fighting infection, reducing anemia, lowering the risk of heart disease, and supporting nervous system function.

Fermented foods contain copious amounts of vitamin C, which our bodies cannot synthesize. Vitamin C plays an essential role in hundreds of metabolic functions: it metabolizes cholesterol, acts as an antioxidant that helps slow aging in cells, and helps boost the immune system. Deirdre Rawlings, a widely published naturopath, maintains that, as opposed to cooked or raw cabbage, cabbage as sauer kraut enables us to absorb three to four hundred times more vitamin C.

Fermented cabbage also contains vitamin K, which helps regulate calcium and blood sugar levels.

PROBIOTICS HAVE HEALING POWERS. While scientists do not fully understand the mechanisms of how bacteria work in our bodies, and how the bacteria we eat support our native bacteria, hundreds of studies have been published documenting the role that *specific* probiotics play in preventing disease. In his book *The Art of Fermentation*, Sandor Ellix Katz notes that "the array of conditions for which probiotic therapy has been found to have some documented and quantifiable measure of success is quite staggering." He cites many studies that document the benefits of probiotic therapies for treating digestive-tract conditions such as diarrhea, inflammatory bowel disease, irritable bowel syndrome, constipation, and even colon cancer. Probiotics can lessen the frequency and length of common colds and upper respiratory symptoms, lower high blood pressure and reduce cholesterol, and reduce anxiety. Leading researchers also believe probiotics might prove effective against new pathogens that doctors have so far not found a way to treat.

Lacto-fermented foods replenish and diversify the bacteria in our bodies and help restore the balance of our good bacteria. Research has shown that the types of bacteria that live in our intestines are largely determined by our dietary habits. Our gut bacteria are a dynamically changing community, so by supplying gut flora with fermented foods, we augment our intestinal communities.

An Easy Solution: Eat Fermented Foods

In other words, eating fermented foods is good for you. Scientists who specialize in research on the human microbiome—the community of microbes within the gut—report that, as a result of what they've learned about bacteria in the body, they've added fermented foods like sauerkraut, kimchi, and yogurt to their diets for the large number of probiotic bacteria in those foods.

Our own anecdotal evidence certainly supports this. Since we've been in business, we've heard literally hundreds of testimonials about the good effects of eating Firefly Kitchens' fermented foods, particularly about the benefits to digestion.

Although probiotics found in lacto-fermented foods are not a panacea, they can be an essential part of a varied healthy diet—and that healthy diet is what we

HOW MUCH CAN I EAT IN A DAY?

Some people eat as little as a tablespoon a day and enjoy improved digestion, while others eat as much as half a cup with every meal. Everybody processes foods differently; learn to listen to your body to know how much to eat.

When you're introducing fermented foods to your diet, start with just a tablespoon at a time. You may experience a bit of gas and bloating at first, but these side effects should diminish as you continue eating them.

want to help you create. This book gives you recipes that will help you eat fermented foods every day and teaches you approaches for integrating these foods into your diet without a lot of extra work.

So turn the page and learn how to feed your gut and help your gut feed you!

Firefly's Top Ten Tips for Better Digestion

1. Enjoy each meal sitting down
Movement signals your body to put energy elsewhere. Digestion requires focused energy.

2. Avoid eating when angry, upset, or under stress
Highly emotional states inhibit proper digestion by activating the "fight or flight" response in the nervous system. This phase prepares the body for action and inhibits the processes necessary for digestion.

3. Avoid screens while eating
Computers, phones, and TVs are a distraction and will zap the true enjoyment out of any meal. Mindless eating means you're not paying attention to how much you are consuming, how fast you're taking it in, or how well you're chewing it.

4. Chew your food!
Think about chewing your food twice as long as you normally do. Digestion is already in progress once your food reaches your mouth. Thorough chewing equals a happy belly.

5. Practice not overeating
Eat until 80 percent full and leave the rest. This may very well be one of the greatest secrets to longevity and vibrant health!

6. Eat early, not late
Make the first meal of the day nourishing one, and avoid eating late at night. We are not designed to digest while we sleep!

7. Move your body every day
Exercise helps digestion by increasing blood flow and oxygen to all of your organs, while strengthening the intestinal muscles. This helps to more efficiently move food through the entire GI system.

8. Get adequate fiber
Fiber is the broom that moves foods through our system. Fruits, veggies, whole grains, and ferments ensure your body is getting what it needs to function properly.

9. Consume healthy fats at every meal
Healthy fats such as coconut oil, avocados, olive oil, and butter from grass-fed cows are satisfying and decrease levels of inflammation within the gut.

10. Eat ferments at every meal!
Fermented foods are rich in lactic acid and digestive enzymes, so eating them equals optimal digestion and optimal health.

Chapter 2:
Making Classic Kraut

IN THIS CHAPTER, learn how simple it is to make a jar of effervescent and crunchy kraut at home. That's how we started—in our kitchens at home. Making jar after jar after jar of kraut, hundreds of jars. And since then, at Firefly Kitchens, we've processed sixty tons of vegetables, a lot of it with our own hands.

As we've learned, fermenting vegetables is a journey of both science and art, a journey that follows time-honored traditions. The science is fermentation, and it takes care of itself. The art is in nurturing the fermentation to achieve the best results possible—every time.

You don't need much to get going—a few very basic tools, some fresh vegetables, pure sea salt, and spices. What follows are detailed how-to instructions and lessons learned—everything from how much salt to use to how long to let the cabbage ferment and what to do when things go wrong.

As you practice making kraut, we encourage you to keep notes on each batch—maybe in the form of a fermentation journal like the ones we've always kept. Each time you make it, take note of what happened when you changed the salt level or fermentation time, fermented at a different temperature, or added a new spice. You'll learn from what you observed and tasted, and discover how you might alter what you do next time.

We encourage you to experiment with other vegetables and spices or adjust the quantities of those we specify. It doesn't take much effort to double the recipes, so you can make the standard recipe and brew a unique batch alongside it. Through practice, documentation, and experimentation, you'll create your own tradition of fermentation.

Basic Tools

BOWL. It should be big enough to comfortably hold 12 cups (3 quarts) of shredded cabbage and have enough room to mix the cabbage vigorously with your hands.

LARGE KNIFE OR FOOD PROCESSOR WITH SLICING BLADES.

JAR. A quart jar with a wide mouth, like a Mason or Ball jar, is easiest to pack cabbage into—you can get your fingers in there—but you can use any quart-size jar you have around, like recycled mayonnaise, peanut butter, or pickle jars. You'll also need a lid that fits the jar; plastic lids are less likely to corrode than metal, but either will work.

WIDE-MOUTH FUNNEL (OPTIONAL). This helps you get the cabbage into the jar without making a big mess, but it's not required. (You can always wipe up the mess!)

WEIGHTS (OPTIONAL). When you make kraut, you'll need some way to keep the cabbage submerged in brine; a weight is one way to do this. Anything small enough to fit in the mouth of the jar and heavy enough to weigh cabbage down will work: a glass coaster, votive candle holder, small glass jar filled with something to make it heavier, or a rock (Julie's favorite). The core of the cabbage works well too.

Basic Ingredients

CABBAGE (AND OTHER VEGETABLES). We prefer organic vegetables, which are grown without pesticides and often have more vivid flavors, but you can make great kraut with conventionally grown vegetables too. Whatever you decide, get the freshest vegetables you can for the best flavor.

We prefer green cabbage. When we were developing our kimchi recipe, we experimented with napa cabbage and didn't get the same crunchy results. It's also been our experience that red cabbage works differently than green cabbage—for example, it doesn't seem to break down as much or as easily when you work in the salt. But go ahead and experiment with these and any variety of cabbage that appeals to you.

SEA SALT. Salt triggers the magic of fermentation, so you want to use the right one. Salt comes either from the sea or salt mines (the source of most of today's salt), which are salt deposits from ancient seas.

Table salt isn't good for fermentation. It's usually highly refined—bleached, stripped of its natural magnesium salts and trace minerals, diluted with anticaking chemicals, and supplemented with iodine. Iodine has bacteria-killing properties, and fermentation relies on bacteria to work. Also, iodized salt can darken the color of kraut, and while it's perfectly edible, you might not like the way it looks.

At Firefly, we always use the Celtic Sea Salt brand, which is far from typical table salt. It's unrefined, full of its natural minerals, and has no additives. If you use another sea salt, make sure it's not iodized, and look for an unrefined salt with its natural color intact—pink, off-white, or gray, for example. The colors are indicators of the minerals present in the salt.

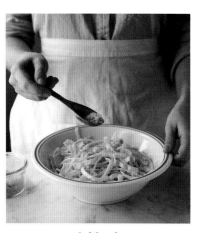

Add salt

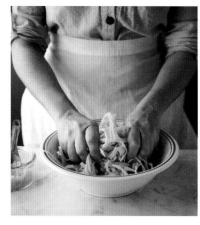

Work the cabbage

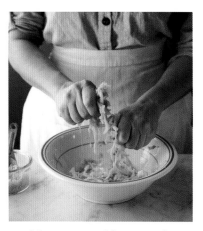

Massage until brine pools

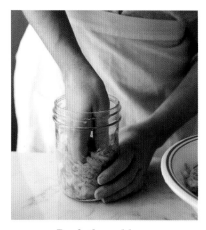

Pack the cabbage

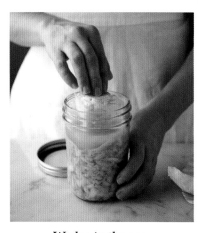

Wedge in the core

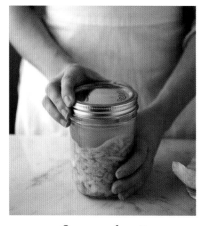

Cover and wait

SPICES. Classic Kraut uses no spices, but all of the other Firefly krauts do—for example, caraway seeds, dried dill, and ground coriander.

Use only fresh, dried spices. Smell yours. Do you smell a distinctive fragrance? If so, they're probably okay; if not, it's time to go shopping. The best way to buy spices is in bulk. That way you can buy small amounts—as little as an ounce at a time—so you use them up before they get stale. It's cheaper that way too!

How to Make Classic Kraut

Classic Kraut is our most basic sauerkraut recipe, our original kraut, and still one of our best sellers. It's kraut plain and simple without any additions like onion, garlic, or hot pepper, so anyone can eat it, including those on healing journeys who've been directed to eat fermented foods. It's the basis for all the other Firefly ferments, which you will learn to make in the next chapter.

Basically, you'll be adding salt to cabbage, massaging and pounding the cabbage to break down its cell walls, packing it into a jar, and then submerging the cabbage in its own brine. While you wait for a week or more, the friendly bacteria that live on the cabbage transform it into vibrant, tangy sauerkraut.

As you embark on your kraut-making journey, follow the directions carefully, like a scientist. But remember that making kraut is also an art, so attend to your senses—touch, sight, smell, taste—and let them guide you as you proceed.

IN A NUTSHELL: STEPS FOR MAKING KRAUT

Once you have made your first batch of kraut, you will be thrilled with the simplicity of the process. Let this serve as your "kraut-making at a glance."

- Clean everything
- Make the brine
- Get the cabbage ready
- Work the cabbage
- Taste for salt
- Pack the cabbage into the jar
- Cover the jar, set it aside . . . and wait
- Taste the kraut and store it
- Preserve the kraut

Clean everything

Cleanliness is important when you make kraut, so start with a clean work space and wash tools and jars in hot, soapy water or put them through the dishwasher. However, keep in mind that folks making kraut a hundred years ago weren't bleaching down their kitchens.

Make the brine

When you make kraut, always taste it before you jar it. Like the three bears' porridge, it should not have too much salt or too little, but a salt level that's just right. It's a challenge to describe for those just starting out how salty is "just right," so the brine recipe below will serve as your baseline.

Mix up some brine and taste it. This is how properly salted cabbage should taste. (As you get some experience, you will begin to develop your palate to taste perfectly salted cabbage without comparing it to brine.)

Also, you will likely need extra brine. Maybe the cabbage is dry (carrots too) from having been in storage at the grocery store or in your fridge a while. Maybe you got tired of massaging the cabbage before there was enough of the salty liquid. Or, during the fermentation process, you might need to top off the jar with brine. Whatever the reason, brine is super easy to make.

You need to remove the chlorine from tap water because chlorine inhibits the growth of bacteria—the very reason it's added to our water supply. If you don't filter your water, you can boil it in an uncovered pot to evaporate the chlorine. Just make sure to cool it to room temperature before you use it so you don't kill the bacteria on the cabbage.

Makes 1 cup brine

1 cup water at room temperature

1¼ teaspoons sea salt

- To make the brine, stir the salt into the water until it dissolves.

Get the cabbage ready

1 head green cabbage (about 2 pounds)

1 tablespoon sea salt

- Peel off any older, discolored outer leaves (don't throw them out!), and rinse the head in cold water.

- Quarter the cabbage and remove the core. (Don't throw the core out either. You may use it and the outer leaves later to help keep the compressed cabbage below the brine when you pack the kraut into the jar.)

- Slice the cabbage into long, thin strips, about ⅛ inch to ¼ inch wide. Make the slices as uniform as possible so the cabbage will ferment evenly. (The thinner the strips, the quicker the cabbage will ferment.) You should have about 12 cups of shredded cabbage. (It's hard to believe that all this cabbage will fit into a quart jar, but it usually does.)

- Put the cabbage into a large bowl and sprinkle it with the salt. You can let the salted cabbage sit for 20 minutes so the salt starts to pull the water from the cabbage, reducing the time you need to work it.

TIP: If your bowl isn't large enough to hold all the cabbage at once, add as much cabbage as it can comfortably hold and a portion of the salt. As you work it, the cabbage will shrink, and you can gradually add the rest of the cabbage and salt.

Work the cabbage

The idea here is to thoroughly mix the salt with the cabbage, which helps to draw the water out, creating a brine. You are also trying to distribute the salt evenly—otherwise, the resulting kraut might be mushy or a dark color. It may still be edible, but you might not like the texture or color.

We like to use our hands to work the salt into the cabbage. Work it hard—massaging, whacking, tossing, turning, mashing, squeezing, beating, and pounding it. Some people like to use a (nonmetallic) pounder, such as a rock or the bottom of a Mason jar. It's a great workout! There's something therapeutic about doing this by hand. (If you've ever kneaded bread, you'll know what we mean.)

It can take 5 to 10 minutes of vigorous massaging and pounding to get a mixture of cabbage and brine. Notice that, as you work the cabbage, it will shrink in volume, and in most cases, the brine will increase in volume. Don't be alarmed if the cabbage mixture has a foamy top layer; that's just a sign of good mixing.

FERMENTATION: BEHIND THE SCENES

That cabbage that you've been working on is covered with bacteria (even after you wash it). And that's a good thing, because it's those bacteria—lactic acid bacteria—that are going to ferment the cabbage and turn it into kraut.

The addition of salt and the massaging helps to break down the cell walls and draw the water out of the cabbage, which creates the brine and starts the fermentation process. This enables the lactic acid bacteria to feed on the starches and sugars released, creating a by-product, lactic acid, the fermenting juice. (Carbon dioxide is also released as a gas.) When you pack the cabbage tightly into the jar and submerge it in brine, this creates the ideal oxygen-free environment that sustains lactic acid bacteria.

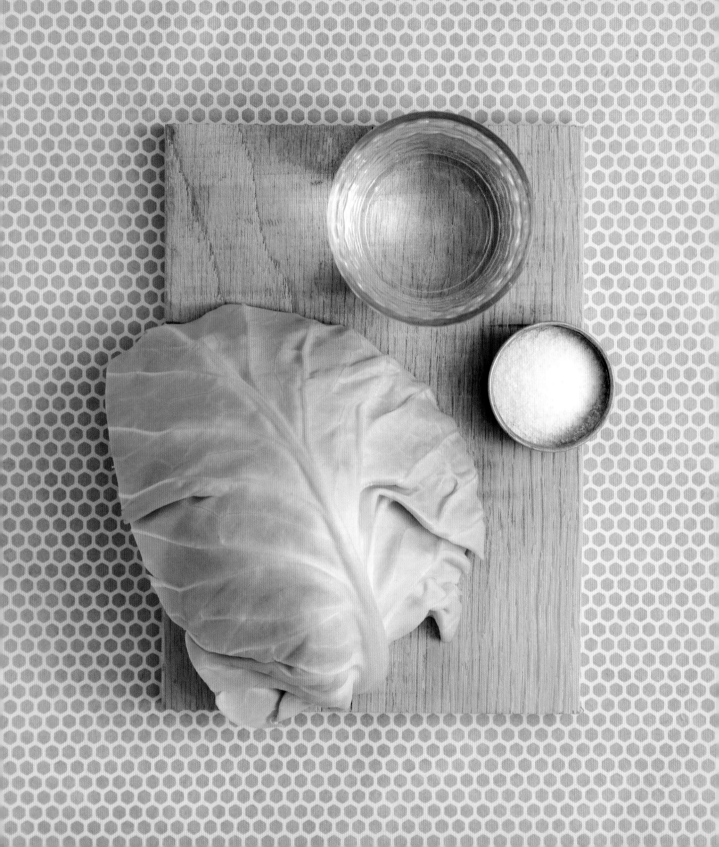

Taste for salt

When the cabbage has shrunk to about half its original volume, and there's a briny, watery base, you know it's time to taste it!

• Taste the cabbage from the bottom of the bowl. It should taste really salty, like you completely oversalted your food or got a mouthful of an ocean wave when you were swimming. Now, taste the saltwater brine you made, and compare. The salt level should taste similar.

• If your cabbage isn't salty enough, add ½ teaspoon of salt to the cabbage, mix it in well, and then taste it again. If it's too salty, add 1 to 2 tablespoons of nonchlorinated water, mix it in well, and then taste. In both cases, add salt or water in these increments until the cabbage is as salty as the brine you made.

Tasting is part of your kraut education, and after making just a few quarts you'll begin to develop a good sense of whether or not the salt level is just right without having to compare it to the saltwater brine you made.

We cannot emphasize enough the importance of using the right amount of salt. Too much salt, and you'll slow the fermentation process to a crawl; too little, and the vegetables might get mushy or moldy. We try to use the least amount required, so we suggest a starting point of 1 tablespoon of salt for every 12 cups of shredded cabbage. However, because the saltiness of the cabbage can vary depending on what kind of salt you use, how carefully or loosely you measure, and other variables, you may need to adjust it using the taste test.

Pack the cabbage into the jar

Your goal here is to protect the compressed cabbage from exposure to air. (The oxygen in the air is what harmful bacteria need to grow.)

• Press the cabbage down into the jar until it's about 2 inches below the rim. Pack it tightly so there are no air pockets. If all of the cabbage won't fit, that's okay. (Sauté up the extra or throw it into a stir-fry.)

• To fill the space between the compressed cabbage and the lid and hold the cabbage under the brine, wedge in the outer leaves and core of the cabbage, or use a weight (see Basic Tools, page 27). (It's likely that you'll have to throw out this top layer of cabbage that's been exposed to the air, but everything tucked in below the brine will be fine.)

- Make sure the brine completely covers the compressed cabbage by about 1 inch, and that it's about 1 inch below the rim of the jar. This provides some buffer space if the gas (carbon dioxide) that the fermentation generates pushes up the cabbage and the brine bubbles out. If there's not enough liquid to cover the cabbage, add as much brine (see Make the brine, page 30) as you need.

Cover the jar, set it aside . . . and wait

Air and light are the enemies of multiplying lactic acid bacteria.

- Screw on the lid until it's just tight, but not screwed down hard. (We call this *finger tight*.) The lid tightened in this way will allow the carbon dioxide to escape; if you screw the lid on too tightly, the gas can't get out, and when you open the jar, the brine and gas will burst out.

- Set the jar out of direct sunlight, but also somewhere you can have the fun of watching it ferment—your kitchen counter might be a good spot. Put the jar on a plate or in a shallow bowl in case the brine leaks out. (This is normal because the brine level can increase as more water is pulled from the cabbage.)

Now it's time for the bacteria to do their work, and for you to watch what happens.

Let the jar sit at room temperature, roughly 64 to 70 degrees F, the optimal temperature for these bacteria. If the temperature is too low, the fermentation will take longer; if it's too warm, the cabbage will ferment faster, but the resulting kraut may be softer.

Watch the brine level. If it drops below the cabbage, press down the cabbage, and top it off with more brine (see Make the brine, page 30). If the lid is bulging even just a little, unscrew it slightly to let the carbon dioxide escape so it doesn't burst out of the jar when you open it.

Taste the kraut and store it

After one week the kraut may be ready to eat, so start tasting. It should taste good to you—tart and crunchy. We prefer to wait 3 to 4 weeks.

- If you taste it and decide it's not ready, let it ferment longer to let the flavors mature. Taste the fermenting kraut weekly until it's as tangy as you want, and make sure the cabbage is completely submerged and has no contact with air before you re-cover the jar.

- If you like the flavor and texture, it's ready to eat. Store it in the fridge to slow the fermentation; the flavors will continue to mature.

There's no hard-and-fast rule about how long you can store kraut. It will continue to ferment slowly in the refrigerator, and the flavors will deepen and mature like a ripening cheese or fine wine (although over time, it may soften, losing its crisp texture). Firefly Kitchens' products, from the time of jarring, have a six-month "Best By" date as a guide to the buyer. But we've opened jars that are more than a year old and they've been perfectly fine.

Preserve the kraut

- Keep the brine level at or above the level of the veggies. Every time you take some out of the jar, push the vegetables back under the brine, keeping them covered as much as possible.

- Be careful not to introduce new bacteria into the kraut because it may cause the ferment to spoil. We always recommend using a clean utensil every time you extract kraut or brine from the jar. No double dipping or eating straight out of the jar!

- Use your senses. If you're skeptical about the jar of kraut you find in the back of fridge, look, smell, and then taste. It will be obvious if something's wrong. (Hopefully you won't have this predicament because you'll be eating your ferments as fast as you can make them.)

- When you use kraut, drain the extra brine back into the jar to protect the kraut that is left inside.

- Bacteria will die if they're heated over 110 degrees F. In some of the recipes in this book, we call for kraut before cooking. In those cases, the kraut contributes its texture and flavor, but to get a good dose of probiotics, we almost always add raw kraut to the dish before serving. In your own cooking, when you serve ferments with hot food, we recommend that you wait until it has cooled slightly before you add the kraut so you keep its probiotic benefits.

KITCHEN EFFICIENCY: BLEND A JAR OF KRAUT IN ADVANCE

Some of the recipes in this book, particularly the desserts, call for mincing small amounts of Classic Kraut—sometimes just a couple of tablespoons. It can be difficult to blend such small amounts and get a smooth, even texture.

Make it easy on yourself. Whirl a couple of cups of kraut in a food processor or blender until it's the consistency of applesauce; stash it in the fridge for instant use later. Some recipes will call for squeezing out any extra brine so it doesn't effect the outcome of the final product as in some breakfasts, dips, and desserts.

What to Do When Things Go Wrong

Here are some problems you may encounter, some explanation of what might have gone wrong, and what you can do about it. But trust your senses here—if a batch of kraut just seems "wrong," throw it out and start over.

The problem	Why it might have happened	What to do about it
White scum on top	The kraut may have been exposed to air.	Skim off the scum, then add more brine or weight the kraut to completely submerge it.
Moldy kraut (Mold is the top reason for bad-smelling sauerkraut.)	Mold is common on the surface of the brine, or on the cabbage or the weight, especially if it's been fermenting for a few weeks. This can occur when the fermentation temperature is too high or the cabbage is exposed to air. It's usually only on the surface.	Scrape the mold off so there is no remaining moldy smell or taste, and make sure to submerge the cabbage in brine. Then you can continue to let it ferment. In our years of fermenting, there have been just a handful of times where mold tainted the whole batch. If that happens to you, just throw it out—and try again.
Soft and mushy kraut	This could result from not using enough salt, salting the cabbage unevenly, a fermentation temperature that was too high, or air pockets because the cabbage wasn't packed tightly enough.	It's perfectly safe to eat—in fact some people like it better.
Slimy kraut, maybe with a thick viscous brine	This can occur when the fermentation temperature was too high or there was not enough salt.	Try letting the kraut ferment longer, and the viscosity might dissipate. If it doesn't, throw it out.
Dark kraut	This could result from using iodized salt, salting the cabbage unevenly, a fermentation temperature that was too high, or the cabbage not being trimmed or washed properly. This can also happen if you store the kraut at too high a temperature or for too long.	Throw it out.
Pink kraut	Yeast is growing on the kraut. It may be caused by too much salt (in which yeast thrive), an uneven distribution of salt, or kraut that was improperly weighted or covered.	Throw it out.

Classic Kraut Favorites

Many recipes in this book use Classic Kraut, but you can also think of it as a basic ingredient, as you would lemon juice or vinegar—a tart, acidic, health-giving alternative with its own unique flavor. So when you read a recipe that calls for vinegar (rice wine, sherry, champagne, balsamic) or lemon, consider Classic Kraut and its brine as an alternative or addition.

Classic Kraut is tangy and crunchy, but with a neutral flavor—even people who say they don't like sauerkraut like it. It's tasty on any kind of sausage, hot dog, or burger, and adds zing to grilled veggies and tofu. Or blend it, for example, with fresh dill and sour cream and serve it over grilled fish.

HERE ARE SOME OF OUR FAVORITE
RECIPES TO GET YOU STARTED:

Classic Kraut Smoothie (page 61)

Steel-Cut Oat Bowl (page 79)

Krauty Kale Caesar (page 116)

Pea and Prosciutto Risotto (page 182)

Sweet and Sauer Chocolate
    Pudding (page 208)

KRAUT WON'T MAKE YOU SICK

If you're concerned that someone might get sick from the kraut you make, you can stop worrying. Fred Breidt, a microbiologist who specializes in vegetable fermentation at the U.S. Department of Agriculture (USDA), doesn't know of a single documented case of food-borne illness from fermented vegetables. "Risky isn't a word I would use to describe vegetable fermentation," he shared with Sandor Ellix Katz. "It's one of the oldest and safest technologies we have." The FDA apparently agrees, because it has rated fermented foods as Generally Recognized as Safe (GRAS).

Fermentation protects against harmful bacteria in two ways. During the first few days, when the lactic acid bacteria are beginning to proliferate, the concentration of salt prevents any harmful bacteria present on fresh produce from growing. Then, as the lactic acid bacteria multiply, they break down the starches and sugars in the food, releasing increasing amounts of lactic acid. This creates an acidic environment that inhibits the growth of harmful bacteria but nourishes lactic acid bacteria, so they multiply vigorously and simply crowd out the pathogens.

Chapter 3:

Making Other Firefly
Kitchens Ferments

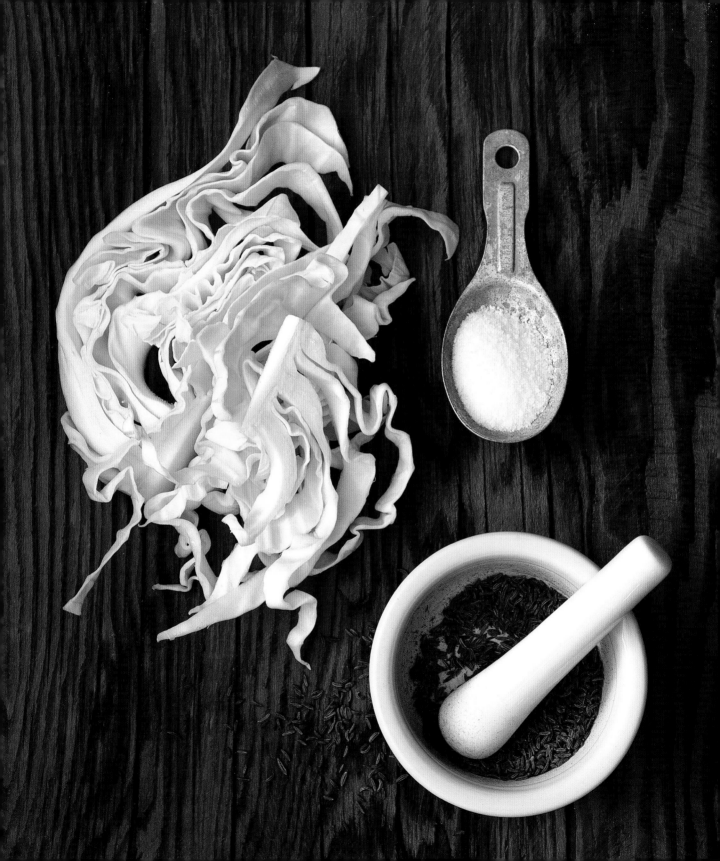

Caraway Kraut

We didn't start making Caraway Kraut until our third year in business—we just weren't sure if our customers would like the distinctive caraway flavor. When we started experimenting, however, it took just one test batch to convince us that Caraway Kraut belonged in Firefly's lineup of fermented foods.

Caraway Kraut contributes its pleasing earthy taste to some of the recipes in this book and also makes a great side dish for grilled meats or mashed potatoes. It's the perfect addition to the classic Reuben (of course) and adds intrigue to potato salads and coleslaws too. Whirl it with fresh avocado for a simple sandwich spread or as a dip for chips and veggies. (The acid does double duty—it adds flavor and keeps the avocado from getting brown.)

Caraway Kraut brine, which results from the fermentation process, is a delicious tonic on its own. For hundreds of years people have been drinking sauerkraut brine to heal ulcers or temper hangovers—it's a well-known Russian remedy—and that inspired us to start bottling and selling the extra brine as our first Tummy Tonic.

Peel off any older, discolored outer leaves from the cabbage, reserving the leaves, and rinse the head. Quarter and core the cabbage, reserving the core. Slice the cabbage into ⅛- to ¼-inch-wide strips. You should have about 12 cups of shredded cabbage.

Put the cabbage in a large bowl and sprinkle it with the salt. Use your hands to thoroughly work the salt into the cabbage. When the cabbage has shrunk to about half its original volume and has generated a briny, watery base, taste it and add more salt or water if necessary. Stir in the caraway seeds, making sure they're evenly distributed throughout the ferment.

Pack the cabbage tightly into a quart jar until it's about 2 inches below the rim, weighing it down with the reserved leaves and core. Make sure the brine completely covers the compressed cabbage by about 1 inch, and that it's about 1 inch below the rim

continued

Makes about 1 quart

1 head green cabbage (about 2 pounds)

1 tablespoon sea salt

2 teaspoons caraway seeds

Now that you have our most basic Classic Kraut under your belt, here are some adaptations, each with its own unique flavor and health benefits. If you don't feel like shredding and massaging all that cabbage and want a slightly more instant gratification, look to the Quick & Simple variations. Of course, all that work and longer fermenting time yields a fuller flavor, so the speedier version won't taste quite the same.

of the jar. Let the jar sit at room temperature, roughly 64 to 70 degrees F, topping the cabbage with more brine if needed. The kraut could be ready to eat after 1 week (or let it ferment longer for a richer taste). Store it in the refrigerator for up to 6 months.

Make It Quick & Simple

Start with 2 cups of your own Classic Kraut, or 1 pound plain unpasteurized sauerkraut from your local market. (You'll find it in the refrigerator case.)

Stir 1 to 1½ teaspoons of crushed caraway seeds into the kraut and mix well. Crush the caraway seeds using a mortar and pestle, rolling pin, or clean coffee grinder. Break them down, but don't crush them to a powder. Crushing them helps the caraway flavor more fully permeate the kraut.

Pack the entire mixture into a jar, and top off with as much Brine (page 30) as needed to cover the kraut.

Let the jar sit at room temperature out of bright light for about a week, and then refrigerate. It's ready to eat; however, the longer you let it ferment, the more fully the flavors will develop.

CARAWAY KRAUT FAVORITES:

Caraway Raita Soother (page 71)

Green Bean Potato Salad (page 119)

Paprika Potatoes (page 158)

Ruby Red Kraut

Our brilliantly colored kraut won a Gold Seal at the Good Food Awards in 2013. People always call it the "beet kraut" due its gorgeous hue, which ranges from a vibrant magenta to a rich, dark red—a gift of the beets and red cabbage. Research suggests that these red pigments (called anthocyanins) have anti-inflammatory and anti-carcinogenic effects, alleviate diabetes, and help control obesity.

Since Ruby Red Kraut has no particular spice, it pairs well with almost anything, and makes a colorful addition to roasts, grilled meats, turkey sandwiches, mashed or baked potatoes, or grain salads. Toss it with fresh greens, dried cherries, sliced apples, candied nuts, and feta cheese for a tasty salad.

Mix the green and red cabbage, carrots, and beets in a large bowl. Add the salt, using your hands to thoroughly work the salt into the vegetables. When the vegetables have shrunk to about half their original volume and have generated a briny, watery base, taste them and add more salt or water if necessary. Mix in the green onions, making sure they're evenly distributed throughout.

Pack the vegetables tightly into a quart jar until they're about 2 inches below the rim, weighing them down with the reserved leaves and core. Make sure the brine completely covers the compressed vegetables by about 1 inch, and that it's about 1 inch below the rim of the jar.

Let the jar sit at room temperature, roughly 64 to 70 degrees F, topping the vegetables with more brine if needed. The kraut should be ready to eat after 1 week (or let it ferment longer for a richer taste). Store it in the refrigerator for up to 6 months.

> **NOTE:** Make sure both kinds of cabbage are shredded as uniformly as possible, so they'll ferment evenly. Reserve any older, discolored outer leaves and the cores to weigh the ferment down in the jar.

Makes about 1 quart

8 cups thinly shredded green cabbage (a bit less than 1½ pounds)

3 cups thinly shredded red cabbage (about ½ pound)

½ cup grated carrot

½ cup peeled and grated beet

4 teaspoons sea salt

⅓ cup thinly sliced green onions, including the green tops

continued

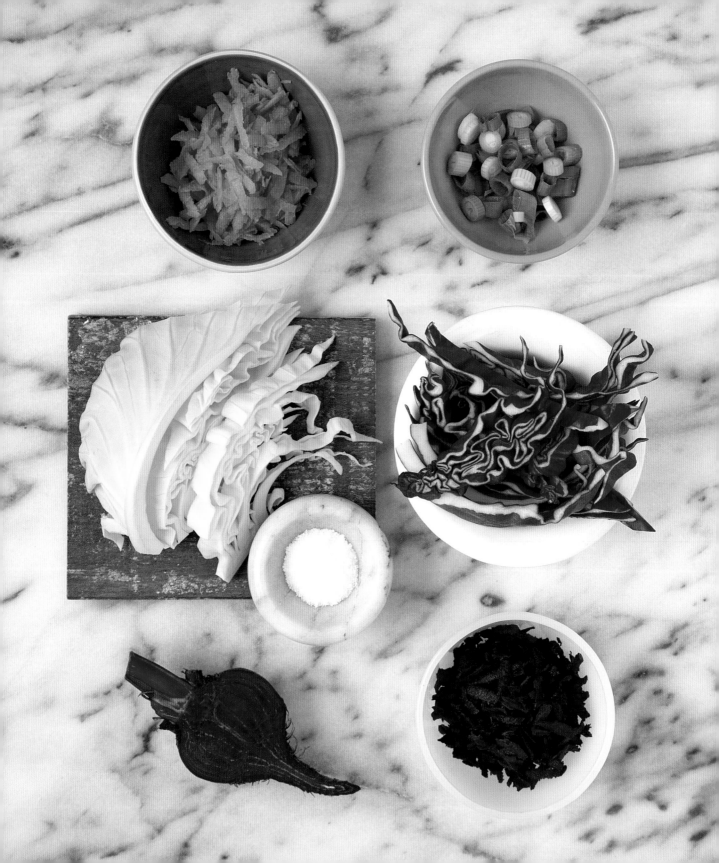

Make It Quick & Simple

Start with 2 cups of your own Classic Kraut, or 1 pound plain unpasteurized sauerkraut from your local market. (You'll find it in the refrigerator case.)

To the kraut, add ¾ cup shredded beets, ¼ cup grated carrot, 1 tablespoon minced green onions, and ¼ teaspoon salt. Mix well. Pack the entire mixture into a jar, and top off with as much Brine (page 30) as needed to cover the vegetables.

Let the jar sit at room temperature out of bright light for about a week, and then refrigerate. It's ready to eat; however, the longer you let it ferment, the more fully the flavors will develop.

> **RUBY RED KRAUT FAVORITES:**
>
> Ruby Red Rush (page 68)
>
> Sun-Dried Tomato Tapenade (page 104)
>
> Pear, Fennel, and Pecan Salad (page 122)
>
> Triple-B Veggie Burgers (page 142)
>
> Scarlet Millet (page 150)
>
> Salmon with Caraway Cream (page 189)

HOW CAN YOU TELL IF FERMENTED VEGGIES IN THE STORE ARE RAW AND UNPASTEURIZED?

Look for raw and unpasteurized ferments in the refrigerated section, and then refer to the label for the words "raw," "alive," "fermented," "cultured," or "unpasteurized." If you don't see those, it won't contain the live probiotics that you're seeking, the important difference between a healthy, nutrient-dense product and one that's not.

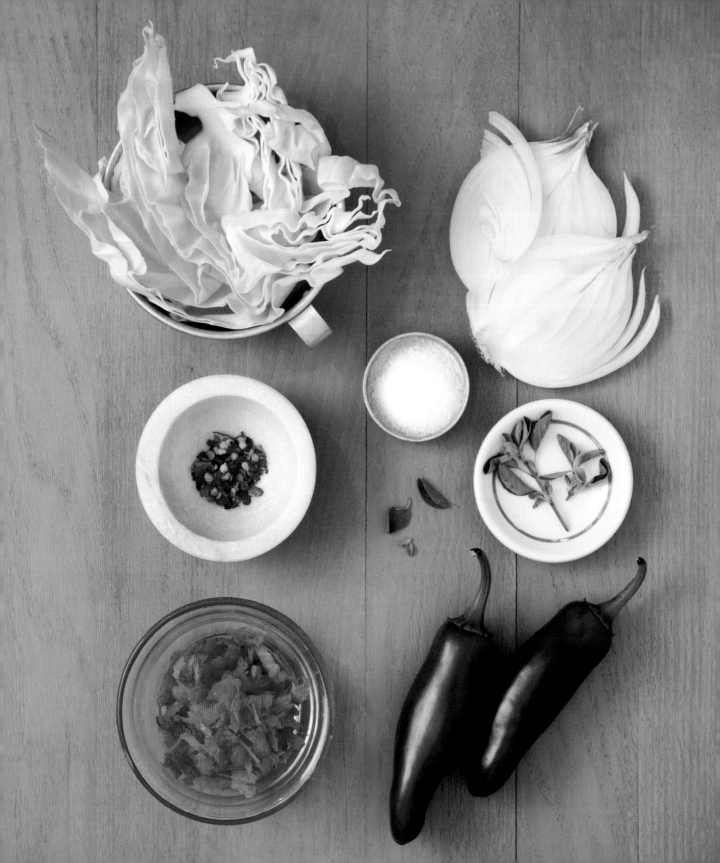

Cortido Kraut

Cortido Kraut, a Good Food Award winner in 2012, is a spin on Salvadoran curtido, a lightly fermented and spicy cabbage relish. Oregano, a prominent herb in Cortido Kraut, is, according to the USDA, a powerful antioxidant with anti-inflammatory benefits.

Cortido Kraut is similar in taste to a mild salsa, yet tangier and crunchier thanks to the fermented cabbage. Serve it anywhere you'd serve a lively salsa: with a big bowl of crispy chips; as a garnish for grilled fish, chicken, or tacos; or stuffed into a burrito. It also makes a great side salad.

We don't add cumin to the Cortido Kraut that we sell, but it adds an intriguing depth of flavor. When you're ready to experiment, try a batch adding two teaspoons of crushed cumin seed and see what you think.

Peel off any older, discolored outer leaves from the cabbage, reserving the leaves, and rinse the head. Quarter and core the cabbage, reserving the core. Slice the cabbage into ⅛- to ¼-inch-wide strips. You should have about 12 cups of shredded cabbage.

Mix the cabbage and carrots in a large bowl. Add the salt, using your hands to thoroughly work the salt into the vegetables. When the vegetables have shrunk to about half their original volume and have generated a briny, watery base, taste them and add more salt or water if necessary. Mix in the onion, jalapeño, oregano, and red pepper flakes, making sure they're evenly distributed throughout.

Pack the vegetables tightly into a quart jar until they're about 2 inches below the rim, weighing them down with the reserved leaves and core. Make sure the brine completely covers the compressed vegetables by about 1 inch, and that it's about 1 inch below the rim of the jar. Let the jar sit at room temperature,

continued

Makes about 1 quart

1 head green cabbage (about 2 pounds)

1 medium carrot, grated (about ⅔ cup)

1 tablespoon sea salt

½ medium onion, thinly sliced (about 1 cup)

2 teaspoons minced jalapeño

1½ teaspoons dried oregano

2 teaspoons red pepper flakes, or more if you want more heat

roughly 64 to 70 degrees F, topping the vegetables with more brine if needed. The kraut should be ready to eat after 1 week (or let it ferment longer for a richer taste). Store it in the refrigerator for up to 6 months.

Make It Quick & Simple

Start with 2 cups of your own Classic Kraut, or 1 pound plain unpasteurized sauerkraut from your local market. (You'll find it in the refrigerator case.)

To the kraut, add ½ cup grated carrots, ¼ cup minced onion, ¼ teaspoon minced jalapeño, 1 teaspoon dried oregano, and ¼ teaspoon red pepper flakes. Mix them in well. Pack the entire mixture into a jar, and top off with as much Brine (page 30) as needed to cover the kraut.

Let the jar sit at room temperature out of bright light for about a week, and then refrigerate. It's ready to eat; however, the longer you let it ferment, the more fully the flavors will develop.

CORTIDO KRAUT FAVORITES:

Limacado Dip (page 99)

Queen Bean Salad (page 121)

Rustic Grilled Cheese (page 138)

Baked Cortido Polenta (page 160)

Cortido Enchiladas (page 185)

Emerald City Kraut

Turmeric and speckles of green kale give Emerald City Kraut its vibrant color. Turmeric is a healing spice with potent anti-inflammatory, digestive, and circulatory benefits. The combination of turmeric, kale, coriander, and dill, as well as billions of probiotics and digestive enzymes, makes Emerald City one of the most nourishing krauts in our lineup.

This kraut is particularly popular with dill pickle lovers. Some devotees will not make tuna salad unless they have this kraut. The coriander adds a fresh, almost citrusy flavor, so Emerald City Kraut is a great addition to plain grains, salads, and most fish.

Here's a trick to cut the kale into the thinnest of slices: cut out the tough center ribs of the kale leaves and discard them. Stack the leaves on top of each other. Roll them up tightly and slice thinly across the rolled-up leaves. This will give you long, thin strips, known in culinary circles as a chiffonade.

Peel off any older, discolored outer leaves from the cabbage, reserving the leaves, and rinse the head. Quarter and core the cabbage, reserving the core. Slice the cabbage into ⅛- to ¼-inch-wide strips. You should have about 12 cups of shredded cabbage.

Mix the cabbage and kale in a large bowl. Add the salt, using your hands to thoroughly work the salt into the vegetables. When the vegetables have shrunk to about half their original volume and have generated a briny, watery base, taste them and add more salt or water if necessary.

Crush the coriander seeds using a mortar and pestle, rolling pin, or clean coffee grinder. Break them down, but don't crush them to a powder. Mix in the crushed coriander, along with the dill, turmeric, and red pepper flakes, to the vegetables, making sure they're evenly distributed throughout.

continued

Makes about 1 quart

1 head green cabbage (about 2 pounds)

½ cup stemmed kale, sliced chiffonade

1 tablespoon sea salt

1½ teaspoons coriander seeds

1 teaspoon dried dill

½ teaspoon ground turmeric

¼ teaspoon red pepper flakes, or more if you want more heat

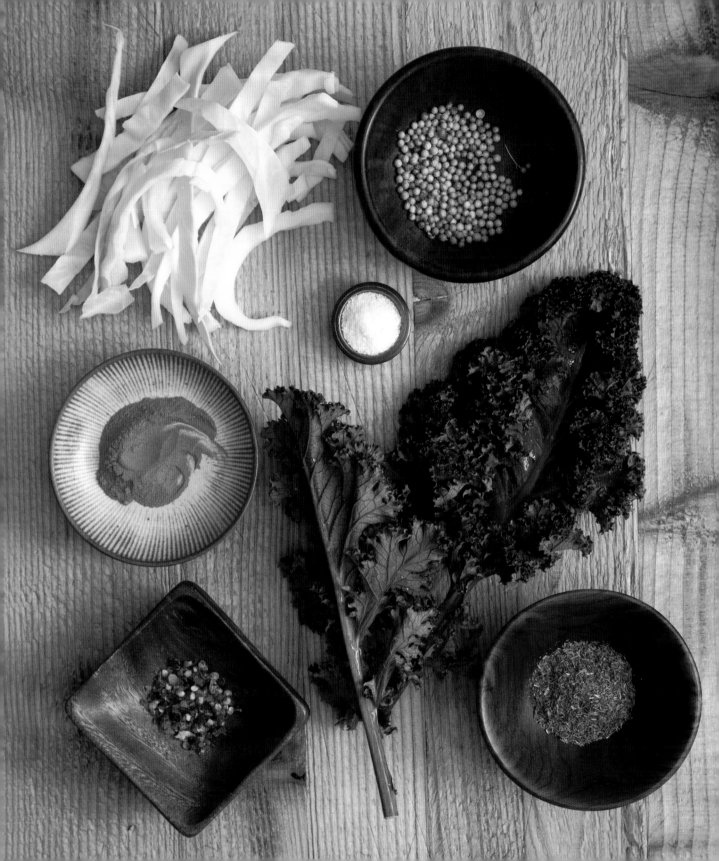

Pack the vegetables tightly into a quart jar until they're about 2 inches below the rim, weighing them down with the reserved leaves and core. Make sure the brine completely covers the compressed vegetables by about 1 inch, and that it's about 1 inch below the rim of the jar. Let the jar sit at room temperature, roughly 64 to 70 degrees F, topping the vegetables with more brine if needed. The kraut should be ready to eat after 1 week (or let it ferment longer for a richer taste). Store it in the refrigerator for up to 6 months.

Make It Quick & Simple

Start with 2 cups of your own Classic Kraut, or 1 pound plain unpasteurized sauerkraut from your local market. (You'll find it in the refrigerator case.)

To the kraut, add ¼ cup stemmed and very thinly sliced kale, ¾ teaspoon crushed coriander seeds, ½ teaspoon dried dill, ¼ teaspoon ground turmeric, and a pinch of red pepper flakes. Mix well. Pack the entire mixture into a jar, and top off with as much Brine (page 30) as needed to cover the vegetables.

Let the jar sit at room temperature out of bright light for about a week, and then refrigerate. It's ready to eat; however, the longer you let it ferment, the more fully the flavors will develop.

> **EMERALD CITY KRAUT FAVORITES:**
>
> Smoked Salmon Mousse (page 96)
>
> Olive Bean Tapenade (page 97)
>
> Emerald City Salad (page 115)
>
> Tri-Way Cabbage Sauté (page 148)

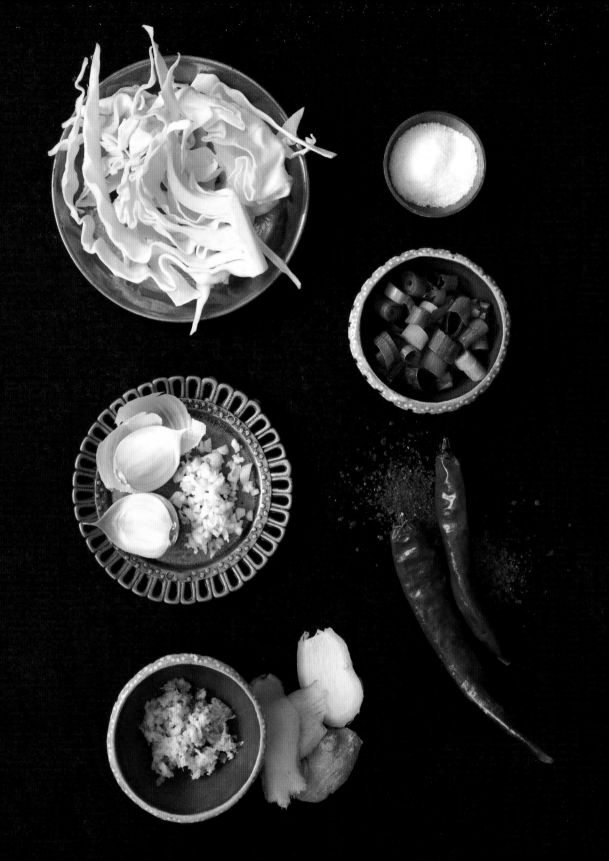

Firefly Kimchi

In 2014, we received our fourth consecutive win at the Good Food Awards with a Gold Seal for Firefly Kimchi, which has always been our best-selling product. Traditional Korean kimchi is made with napa cabbage, daikon, carrots, and Korean peppers, along with a mixture of fish sauce or shrimp paste. Rather than competing with this beloved kimchi, we aimed to offer a pungent, healthy alternative with a similar flavor, omitting the fish sauce and shrimp paste so vegetarians could enjoy it as well. Our early recipe testers picked the green cabbage versions hands down over the napa cabbage batches.

Firefly Kimchi adds a warm ginger and garlic sparkle to whole grains, sautéed greens, or your favorite meats. Mix it into a stir-fry or eat it with eggs instead of ketchup or salsa. Whirl it with cream cheese, hummus, or sour cream to make a flavorful sauce or dip. The ways to enjoy this fantastically flavored food are endless.

Peel off any older, discolored outer leaves from the cabbage, reserving the leaves, and rinse the head. Quarter and core the cabbage, reserving the core. Slice the cabbage into ⅛- to ¼-inch-wide strips. You should have about 12 cups of shredded cabbage.

Put the cabbage in a large bowl and sprinkle it with the salt. Use your hands to thoroughly work the salt into the cabbage. When the cabbage has shrunk to about half its original volume and has generated a briny, watery base, taste it and add more salt or water if necessary. Mix in the green onions, Korean red pepper, garlic, and ginger, making sure they're evenly distributed throughout.

Pack the cabbage tightly into a quart jar until it's about 2 inches below the rim, weighing it down with the reserved leaves and core. Make sure the brine completely covers the compressed cabbage by about 1 inch, and that it's about 1 inch below the rim

continued

Makes about 1 quart

1 head green cabbage (about 2 pounds)

1 tablespoon sea salt

3 tablespoons thinly sliced green onions, including the green tops

1 tablespoon coarsely ground Korean red pepper

2 teaspoons minced garlic

1 teaspoon minced fresh ginger

Korean red pepper (*gochugaru* in Korean) has a more sophisticated flavor than red pepper flakes—slightly smoky and sweet, with a peppery heat. Its deep-red color contributes to the distinctive color of Firefly Kimchi.

Look for 100 percent coarsely ground Korean red pepper, steering clear of brands that contain salt (because you want to control the salt in your fermentation); from our experience about a third of them do. You can find Korean red pepper at Asian food markets or online from many sources, including Amazon.com. If you can't readily get Korean red pepper, you can substitute a pinch of cayenne and 2 teaspoons red pepper flakes, but your kraut won't achieve the unique flavor and color that Korean red pepper delivers.

of the jar. Let the jar sit at room temperature, roughly 64 to 70 degrees F, topping the cabbage with more brine if needed. The kimchi should be ready to eat after 1 week (or let it ferment longer for a richer taste). Store it in the refrigerator for up to 6 months.

Make It Quick & Simple

Start with 2 cups of your own Classic Kraut, or 1 pound plain unpasteurized sauerkraut from your local market. (You'll find it in the refrigerator case.)

To the kraut, add 1 tablespoon minced green onion, 2 teaspoons Korean red pepper, 1 teaspoon minced garlic, and ½ teaspoon minced ginger. Mix them in well. Pack the entire mixture into a jar, and top off with as much Brine (page 30) as needed to cover the kraut.

Let the jar sit at room temperature out of bright light for about a week, and then refrigerate. It's ready to eat; however, the longer you let it ferment, the more fully the flavors will develop.

FIREFLY KIMCHI FAVORITES:

Kimchi Kick-Start Breakfast (page 89)

Firefly Kimcheese (page 95)

PB Chi Spread (page 105)

Kimchi Coleslaw (page 120)

Kimchi'd Mac and Cheese (page 179)

Yin Yang Carrots

Crisp, piquant, and gingery, Yin Yang Carrots will excite even the pickiest of eaters. We won our first Good Food Award in 2011 with this culinary treat. And for good reason. They're such a crowd-pleaser that we always head to the farmers' markets equipped with extra jars. Kids love them too—some parents say this is the only vegetable they can get their kids to eat. Years ago, we saw an adorable two-year-old have a meltdown because her mom couldn't get the lid off the jar fast enough for her little one, who had gobbled up three sample cups.

Of all of our ferments, Yin Yang Carrots are the most versatile, adapting well to the cuisines of many cultures. Tuck them into fresh spring or sushi rolls, blend them into hummus, toss them with salads and slaws, or scatter them on nachos. Try whirling them with olive oil and a dash of sesame oil, hot sauce, and tamari for a flavorful salad dressing. Of course you can always eat them plain—they make a spirited side salad or snack.

We always use organic carrots because they tend to be more flavorful; however, you can make this recipe with conventionally grown carrots too. We use orange carrots, but any color of carrot will work, including yellow, purple, and white. Note that mixing carrots of different colors may not result in the vivid colors of a single-color batch.

Put the carrots in a large bowl and sprinkle them with the salt. Use your hands to thoroughly work the salt into the carrots. When the carrots have shrunk down to about half their original volume and have generated a briny, watery base, taste them and add more salt or water if necessary. Add the ginger, starting with 2 teaspoons, making sure it's evenly distributed throughout. Taste and add the additional ginger if a stronger flavor is desired.

Pack the carrots tightly into a quart jar until they're about 2 inches below the rim, weighing them down with a weight.

> Before grating, scrub the carrots of any visible dirt. Grate them on the large holes of a handheld grater. Using the grating blade of a food processor will yield pieces that are too small, and they will get smaller when you massage and pound the salted carrots.

Makes about 1 quart

8 cups coarsely grated carrots (about 2 pounds)

6 teaspoons sea salt

2 to 4 teaspoons grated fresh ginger (leave the peel on if you'd like)

continued

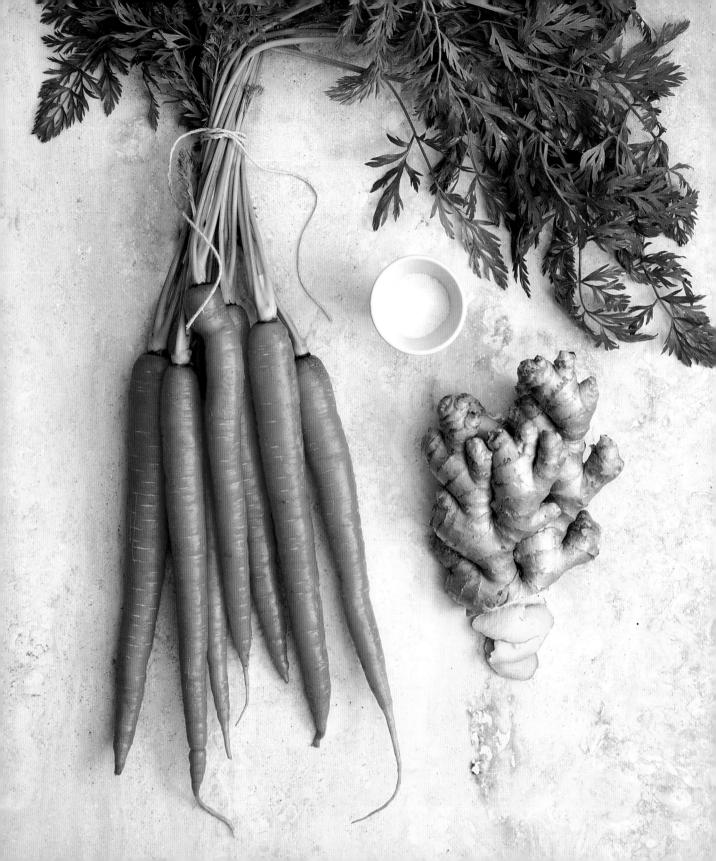

Make sure the brine completely covers the compressed carrots by about 1 inch, and that they're about 1 inch below the rim of the jar. Let the jar sit at room temperature, roughly 64 to 70 degrees F, topping the carrots with more brine if needed. The carrots should be ready to eat after 1 week (or let them ferment longer for a richer taste). Store them in the refrigerator for up to 6 months.

YIN YANG CARROT FAVORITES:

Yin Yang Smoothie (page 65)

Curried Carrot Quinoa Salad (page 114)

Yin Yang Yams (page 152)

Carrot Bars with Carrot Cream Frosting (page 205)

Yin Yang Carrot Balls (page 207)

Chapter 4:
Smoothies & Drinks

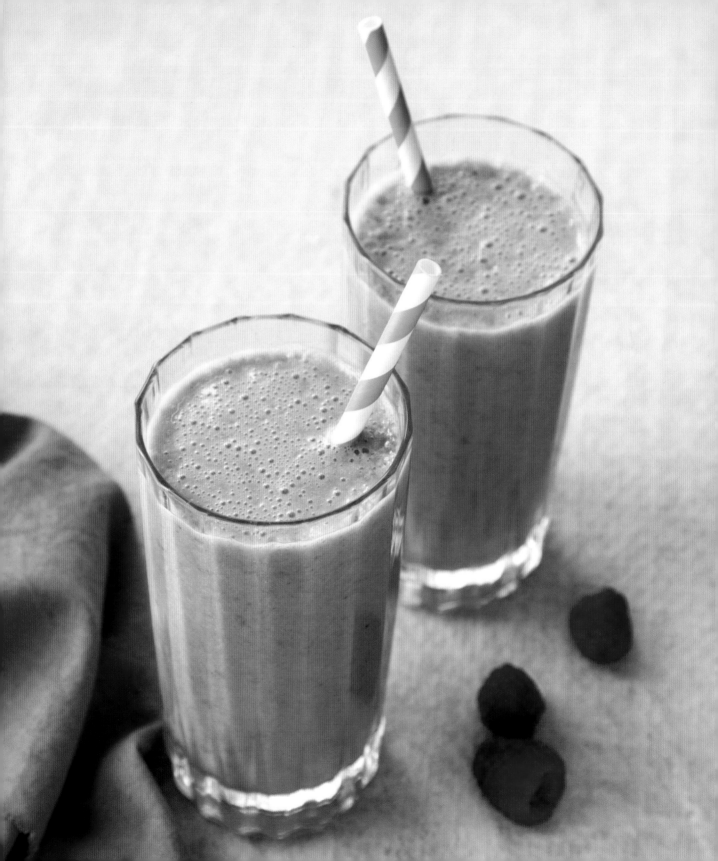

Classic Kraut Smoothie

If you're not sure how the tangy flavor of kraut will work in a smoothie, start with this simple recipe and your taste buds will surely warm up to the idea. The kraut flavor is barely noticed—perfect for sharing with kids and those with less adventurous palates.

The kraut adds a slightly tart zip that enlivens the flavors of the fruits, but you don't even taste it. Rather, the sweetness of the banana and antioxidant-rich blueberries is what stands out. The almond milk provides protein and a nice creamy, nondairy base.

Put together this simple smoothie in minutes with fresh or frozen fruit, and dress it up with yogurt, hemp seeds, protein powder, cod liver oil, coconut oil, or any other smoothie supplement you like.

Put all the ingredients in a blender and whirl until smooth. Drink right away.

KRAUT IN SMOOTHIES? THAT'S CRAZY!

Almost any combination of fruit or veggies can accommodate a small dose of kraut, boosting the drink's nutritional value without significantly altering its flavor. These kraut-filled smoothies are filling and nourishing, the simplest and best-tasting way to jump-start your morning or often light enough to drink as an appetizer before dinner. Our blends are a great way to reduce your sugar intake and pack more vegetables into your day.

Makes 2 to 3 servings

1 medium banana

1 cup fresh or frozen
   blueberries or raspberries

1 apple, nectarine, or pear,
   quartered and cored

¼ cup Classic Kraut (page 29)

1 cup almond milk or milk of
   your choice

Card-o-Nut Smoothie

Creamy, rich, and aromatic—like an Indian spiced shake—this smoothie is a satisfying option for those who are wary of drinking their kraut. Sesame seeds are a great source of calcium, and the cardamom may help alleviate stomach cramps and stimulates the flow of bile, which aids in the metabolism of fats.

Soaking the almonds, dates, cardamom, and fennel seeds in water the night before you whip up the smoothie makes the flavors more robust and the almonds easier to digest. A shot of cooled espresso, or a little cold brewed coffee or iced black tea, adds to the energizing nature of the ingredients.

Makes 1 to 2 servings

¼ teaspoon cardamom seeds (add more if you love cardamom)

1 tablespoon fennel seeds

10 almonds

4 pitted dates

½ cup water

2 cups milk (dairy, rice, almond, coconut, or other)

2 tablespoons sesame seeds

1 tablespoon coconut oil

⅓ cup Classic Kraut (page 29)

Crush the cardamom and fennel seeds using a mortar and pestle, rolling pin, or clean coffee grinder. Break them down, but don't crush them to a powder.

Put the crushed seeds, almonds, dates, and water in a small bowl or jar to soak, covered, on the counter overnight. In the morning, pour the seed mixture, including the soaking water, into a blender and whirl until smooth. Add the milk, sesame seeds, coconut oil, and kraut. Whirl until smooth, about 30 seconds. Drink right away.

Banana Coconut Smoothie

Peanut butter, coconut, and bananas—need we say more? This smoothie is kid and picky-eater approved. Protein-rich and loaded with potassium, good fats, fiber, and antioxidants, it's a great way to sneak some fermented foods into your morning meal or afternoon snack. Enjoy it pre- or postworkout to give your body a nourishing boost.

Adding a bit of chocolate syrup—or, for adults, even a shot of Baileys!—makes the smoothie even more of a treat.

Put all the ingredients in a blender and whirl until smooth. Drink right away.

HOW TO FREEZE OVERRIPE BANANAS

Peel the banana, slice it, put the slices in a ziplock bag, and pop the bag in the freezer for up to four months. This is a great way to make use of overripe bananas, chill a smoothie, or thicken it.

Makes 2 to 3 servings

1 large banana

2 to 3 tablespoons unsweetened dried coconut

2 tablespoons peanut butter or almond butter

¼ cup Classic Kraut (page 29)

1 cup milk (dairy, rice, almond, coconut, or other)

1 tablespoon coconut oil (optional)

2 tablespoons hemp seeds (optional)

1 to 2 teaspoons honey (optional)

Kimchi Gazpacho Drink

"Oh, wow" is what everyone says when they try this savory blend of kraut and veggies, gazpacho in a glass. Sweet, spicy, and cooling, it makes a wonderful addition to just about any of the savory breakfasts in the following chapter, or serve it as a refreshing summer drink. You really have to try it to believe it, but we think you'll love this adventurous combination. Don't hesitate to add more kimchi for a richer, stronger flavor or more honey to mellow it out.

Makes 2 to 3 servings

1 cup water

¼ cup Firefly Kimchi (page 53)

10 cherry tomatoes, or 1 large tomato

1 stalk celery, chopped

½ medium cucumber, peeled and roughly chopped

½ medium red bell pepper, chopped

Juice of 2 small limes (about 2 to 3 tablespoons)

¼ cup fresh cilantro

1 to 2 teaspoons honey

Pinch of salt and freshly ground black pepper

Put all the ingredients in a blender and whirl until smooth. Drink right away.

Yin Yang Smoothie

High in B vitamins, vitamin C, beta-carotene, and essential fatty acids, this smoothie makes for an ultra-nutritious start to any day. If you have a powerful blender, you can skip the grating and mincing.

A dash of pumpkin pie spice is all you need to give this vibrant orange smoothie festive notes reminiscent of your favorite holiday treat. It tastes great with the addition of ½ cup of cooked yam, sweet potato, or pumpkin.

Put the water and grated carrots in a blender and whirl until the carrots break down into a pulp, about 30 seconds. Add the Yin Yang Carrots, ginger, and dates, and whirl for another 30 seconds. Add the orange, lemon juice, and cashews and whirl until smooth. Drink right away.

Makes 2 to 3 servings

2 cups water

2 medium carrots, grated

½ cup Yin Yang Carrots (page 55)

½ teaspoon minced fresh ginger (optional)

2 to 3 pitted dates, minced

1 small orange, peeled and chopped

1 tablespoon freshly squeezed lemon juice

¼ cup cashews, chopped

Mango Lassi

Lassis are an Indian drink used to enhance digestion before a meal and to cool and refresh the body during the heat of summer. We've added Classic Kraut to a traditional recipe, balancing the sweetness of the mango with the bright flavors of the kraut.

Make the lassi dairy-free by using hemp, rice, or nut milk in place of the yogurt. Fresh ginger or mint brings great flavor and adds to the cooling effect of the drink. Spices like cardamom and cinnamon can enhance its digestive benefits.

If you can't find ripe mangoes at your local grocery, canned or frozen mangoes will work well instead—or substitute another tropical fruit, such as pineapple or papaya.

Makes 1 to 2 servings

1 medium mango, halved, pitted, and peeled

1 cup plain or vanilla yogurt

¼ cup Classic Kraut (page 29)

Put all the ingredients in a blender and whirl until smooth. Drink right away.

IS SAUERKRAUT A BETTER SOURCE OF PROBIOTICS THAN YOGURT?

Naturally fermented yogurt and sauerkraut are both good ways to get probiotics, but sauerkraut is a great alternative for those who can't tolerate dairy. Also, many yogurts are sweetened with sugar or artificial sweeteners that compromise the benefits of the probiotics.

We believe that by consuming a wide variety of fermented foods, including kraut, yogurt, miso, kombucha, and more, you will increase the strains of beneficial bacteria to nourish your gut.

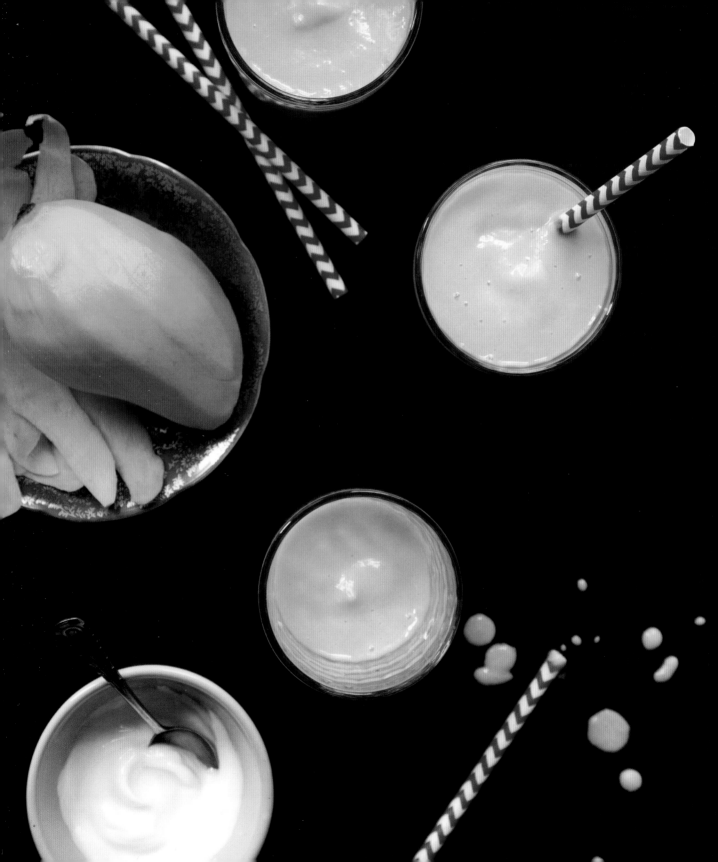

Ruby Red Rush

Considered by many to be one of the most healing and nourishing foods, beets are a fantastic addition to your morning meal. High in folate and potassium, beets have been shown to promote cardiovascular health by protecting against coronary heart disease and stroke. They're also well known for supporting the immune system, promoting liver health, and aiding in natural detoxification processes.

Mixed with strawberries, apples, and fresh ginger, the often powerful flavor of beets becomes mellow and earthy-sweet.

Makes 2 to 3 servings

1 cup water

1 medium carrot, grated

½ small beet, peeled and diced

1 small apple, quartered and cored

1 cup fresh or frozen strawberries or raspberries

⅓ cup Ruby Red Kraut (page 43)

1 cup cherry, cranberry, or apple juice

½ teaspoon minced fresh ginger

1 teaspoon freshly squeezed lemon or lime juice

Put the water, carrot, beet, and apple in a blender and whirl until the vegetables and fruit break down into a pulp, about 30 seconds. (Add a few tablespoons of extra water if the mixture is too dry to blend.) Add the strawberries, kraut, cherry juice, ginger, and lemon juice, and whirl until the mixture is smooth, about 1 minute. Drink right away.

Creamy Cortido Smoothie

Creamy and completely savory, this smoothie is an unexpected and unique treat for the adventurous drinker. Avocado gives it a beautifully smooth consistency, and the citrus juice balances the heat. Enjoy this smoothie as is for a savory breakfast, or add a shot of your favorite spirits to make a great cocktail—Bloody Marys have never been so healthy!

Put all the ingredients except for the salt and pepper in a blender and whirl until smooth. Season to taste with salt and pepper. Drink right away.

CREAMY SMOOTHIES

If you like your smoothies extra creamy, try adding any of the following: banana, avocado, nut butter, silken tofu, coconut cream or butter, yogurt or kefir, or soaked chia seeds.

Makes 2 to 3 servings

⅓ cup Cortido Kraut (page 47)

2 medium carrots, grated

1 medium cucumber, peeled and roughly chopped

1 large tomato, or 8 cherry tomatoes

1 medium avocado, halved, pitted, and peeled

1 cup water

1 tablespoon freshly squeezed lemon or lime juice

1 tablespoon fresh parsley (optional)

3 to 6 dashes of your favorite hot sauce (optional)

Salt and freshly ground black pepper

Emerald City Smoothie

The sweetness of the fruit in this smoothie balances out the vegetable flavors, making it a tasty way to add greens to your morning meal.

Celery, fennel, cucumber, and spinach bring vitamins A, C, and K; folate and magnesium; and antioxidants and anti-inflammatory nutrients to the mix. Apples and dates offer additional fiber and nutrients. Add a handful of frozen berries for an even sweeter flavor or a banana for a creamier texture. You could also omit the fruit entirely for a savory, cleansing drink.

Makes 2 to 3 servings

1 cup water

1 stalk celery, chopped

½ medium fennel bulb, chopped (about 1 cup)

½ medium cucumber, peeled and chopped

1½ cups loosely packed spinach leaves

¼ cup Emerald City Kraut (page 49)

1 apple, quartered and cored

1 to 2 pitted dates (optional)

2 teaspoons minced fresh ginger (optional)

Put the water, celery, fennel, cucumber, and spinach in a blender and whirl until the vegetables break down into a pulp, about 30 seconds. (Add a few tablespoons of extra water if the mixture is too dry to blend.) Add the kraut, apple, dates, and ginger, and whirl until the mixture is smooth, about 1 minute. Drink right away.

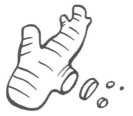

Caraway Raita Soother

Raita is a yogurt-based Indian condiment served alongside spicy foods; the cooling properties of cucumber and yogurt help calm the palate and balance the heat. This smoothie achieves the same cooling effect with a blend of yogurt, cucumber, Caraway Kraut, and fresh herbs. Serve it as an accompaniment to a spicy meal or enjoy it on its own for breakfast or as a cooling postworkout refresher.

Add hemp seeds or an avocado, which are both great sources of healthy fats, for a more filling drink. Kefir, a fermented dairy beverage, works well in place of the yogurt if you want to increase your probiotic intake for the day.

Put all the ingredients, starting with ¼ cup of the water, in a blender and whirl until smooth. If the smoothie is too thick, add water ¼ cup at a time until it's the consistency you want. Drink right away.

Makes 2 to 3 servings

¼ to ½ cup water

⅓ cup Caraway Kraut (page 41)

1 medium cucumber, peeled and chopped

1 cup plain yogurt

1 to 2 tablespoons chopped fresh mint

1 teaspoon freshly squeezed lime juice

1 cup loosely packed spinach leaves (optional)

1 tablespoon chopped fresh cilantro (optional)

Grapefruit Tonic

In Chinese medicine, grapefruit is believed to benefit the stomach and balance the stomach chi. Rounding out the function and flavor of this digestive tonic are cumin and fennel, which are calming to the digestive system. We suggest using whole seeds rather than preground powders.

We use grapefruit juice because it's easier, but a whole, peeled grapefruit works well too. If you choose to use a whole grapefruit, remove the spongy white pith and the seeds, which have a bitter taste. To get the consistency you want, you may also need to add water—or sparkling water for a bubbly beverage.

Makes 1 to 2 servings

1 teaspoon cumin seeds

1 teaspoon fennel seeds

2 cups unsweetened grapefruit juice

2 tablespoons Classic Kraut (page 29)

2 to 3 teaspoons honey

Crush the cumin and fennel seeds using a mortar and pestle, rolling pin, or clean coffee grinder. Break them down, but don't crush them to a powder.

Put the crushed seeds into a blender. Add the grapefruit juice, kraut, and honey, and whirl until smooth. Drink right away, straight up or over ice.

NATURALLY SWEET

Of course, fruit's *the* natural sweetener, but if you're looking for a touch more, here are our favorites: honey, maple syrup, molasses, coconut syrup, and dates.

Lime Sunshine Drink

Legends say that early sailors and explorers kept sauerkraut on their ships because it lasted longer than fresh vegetables during months of voyage, and they later learned it helped prevent scurvy. Limes were also added to the sailors' rations to prevent the same disease. Together in this citrusy drink, sauerkraut and limes complement each other well.

Sweetened by a whole orange, this drink's flavor is reminiscent of tart, pulpy lemonade, although someone with a discriminating palate will notice the touch of kraut. Enjoy it plain on a hot summer day, serve it with a splash of champagne as a spruced-up mimosa, or add some seltzer water and perhaps a shot of rum.

Put all the ingredients in a blender and whirl until smooth. Drink right away.

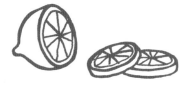

Makes 1 to 2 servings

½ cup water

¼ cup Classic Kraut (page 29)

1 large orange, peeled and roughly chopped

Juice of 2 small limes (about 2 to 3 tablespoons)

4 ice cubes

2 teaspoons honey or maple syrup (optional)

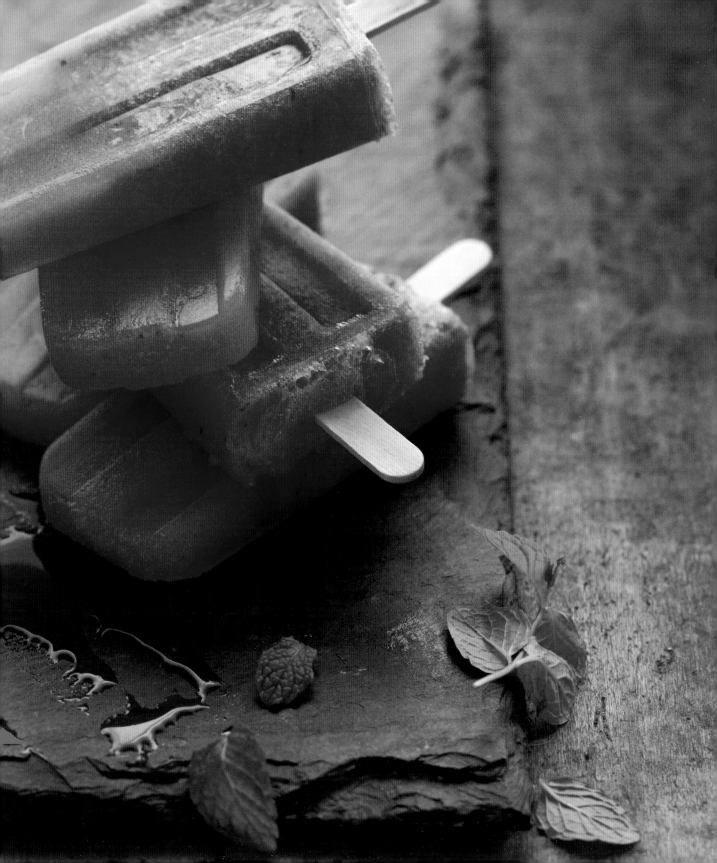

Watermelon Tonic

Finicky eaters won't even notice the kraut in this tonic—it's masked behind the sweet combination of watermelon and strawberries. You can leave the strawberries out for a drink with the pure flavor of watermelon.

Freeze the tonic in small paper cups or Popsicle molds for a special treat on a hot sunny day—in this form, the kids won't think twice about devouring the probiotic-rich concoction. For an adult crowd, accent the sweet summer flavors with fresh mint and a shot of vodka to make an incredible summer cocktail.

Put all the ingredients in a blender and whirl until smooth. Drink right away.

Makes 2 to 3 servings

2 cups diced seedless
  watermelon

1 cup water

½ cup Classic Kraut
  (page 29)

1 cup strawberries, fresh
  or frozen

2 mint leaves, chopped
  (optional)

Chapter 5:
Morning Meals

Firefly Fresh Fruit Bowl **78**

Steel-Cut Oat Bowl **79**

Cardamom Chia
Breakfast Bowl **80**

Kraut over Kitchari **82**

Not Your Mama's Frittata **85**

Latkes with Crème Fraîche
Kraut Sauce **86**

Kimchi Kick-Start Breakfast **89**

Breakfast Burritos
3 Krauty Ways **90**

Firefly Fresh Fruit Bowl

This looks and tastes like a traditional fruit salad, but hidden in each bite is a blast of good bacteria—and vegetables!

For a fancy brunch, an elegant way to present this recipe is to make a yogurt parfait. Mix the kraut and yogurt, then toss all the other ingredients together (except for the almonds) in a separate bowl. To serve, alternate layers of the yogurt and fruit mixtures in individual glasses or a glass bowl (so you can see the layers), garnished with the almonds or granola. If there's any left over, whirl it up into a smoothie with a little extra yogurt for a treat later in the day.

Makes 4 servings

⅓ cup Classic Kraut (page 29)

2 medium bananas, sliced

1 medium apple, cored, and diced

Zest of 1 orange (optional)

1 medium orange, peeled and diced

1 medium nectarine, diced

½ cantaloupe or other melon, seeded and cut into bite-size pieces

2 small fresh apricots, pitted and diced

1 cup Greek yogurt

2 tablespoons unsweetened dried coconut

¼ teaspoon ground cinnamon

2 tablespoons finely minced fresh mint (optional)

Honey, for sweetening

2 tablespoons slivered almonds or granola, for garnish

Take the kraut out of the jar with a clean fork, letting any extra brine drain back into it. Mince the kraut, and mix it in a large bowl with all the remaining ingredients except for the honey and almonds. Taste the fruit; if it's too tart, add honey to your liking. Garnish with the almonds and eat immediately, or chill for up to 3 hours.

> **NOTE:** We change up the fruit combination according to the seasons. It's nice to have a variety of flavors, colors, and textures.

Steel-Cut Oat Bowl

Make a big batch of these oats at the beginning of the week and have a quick and simple healthy breakfast option all week long. Or make some over the weekend for a casual breakfast with family or friends. The chewy texture of steel-cut oats, the crunch of nuts, and the sweetness of the fruit creates a delicious balance. The Classic Kraut brightens it up without overpowering the sweet, nutty notes.

Soaking the oats overnight makes them easier to digest and decreases the cooking time. Adding a fat, whether coconut oil or butter, slows down the absorption of the carbohydrates and helps keep your blood sugar level steady so you feel satisfied longer. (This solves the frequent complaint of feeling hungry just a couple of hours after eating a bowl of oats.)

You can also serve the oats plain and let people add their own toppings. Serve the plain oats in bowls and set out little dishes of nuts, dried fruit, coconut, coconut oil, beets, and minced kraut. Bring the maple syrup to the table and let everyone take it from there. You could add even more toppings, such as sliced fresh fruit, yogurt, or a dusting of cinnamon.

Put the oats in a large pot and add 8 cups of water. Cover the pot and let the oats sit at room temperature for at least 6 hours, or up to overnight. In the morning, thoroughly drain the oats.

Put the drained oats and 3 cups of water in a large pot over medium heat, and bring the water to a boil. Reduce the heat and simmer, stirring occasionally, until the oats are soft and the water is absorbed, about 10 minutes. Remove the pot from the heat, and mix in the cashews, cherries, coconut, coconut oil, and beets.

Take the kraut out of the jar with a clean fork, letting any extra brine drain back into it, and mince the kraut. Serve the oats with the minced kraut on top (or mix it in), and drizzle the maple syrup to taste over the top.

NOTE: If you don't have time to soak the oats (or you forgot!), no problem. Bring 6 cups of water to a boil and stir in 2 cups of steel-cut oats. When the water returns to a boil, lower the heat and simmer, uncovered, stirring every few minutes, until the oats are soft and chewy, 20 to 30 minutes.

Makes 4 servings

- 2 cups steel-cut oats
- 11 cups water, divided
- 1 cup cashews, walnuts, or almonds, finely chopped
- ½ cup dried cherries or cranberries, chopped
- 3 tablespoons dried, unsweetened coconut
- 4 to 8 tablespoons coconut oil or butter
- ½ cup finely shredded raw beets (optional)
- ½ cup Classic Kraut (page 29)
- 2 to 6 tablespoons maple syrup, for serving (optional)

Cardamom Chia Breakfast Bowl

Chia seeds were a significant part of Aztec and Mayan diets—and with good reason. They're a rich source of omega-3 fatty acids and high in fiber. In fact, you only have to eat two tablespoons to get ten grams of daily fiber. Chia seeds are also said to help decrease inflammation, lower cholesterol, and help regulate blood sugar.

This very simple breakfast, with its tapioca pudding–like texture, will quickly become a favorite treat. Soaking the chia seeds overnight helps make them more digestible and meld the flavors of the dates and spices. If dates are not your thing, dried apricots, cherries, or raisins are a good substitute.

Convert this into a healthful dessert by stirring in a little maple syrup and topping the pudding with whipped cream.

Makes 4 to 8 servings

¼ teaspoon cardamom seeds

4 pitted dates, finely chopped

1 cup chia seeds

1 teaspoon ground cinnamon

4 cups almond milk or milk of your choice

½ cup Classic Kraut (page 29)

1 cup roughly chopped pecans (optional)

¼ cup unsweetened dried coconut flakes (optional)

Pinch of salt

Crush the cardamom seeds. Put the cardamom seeds, dates, chia seeds, and cinnamon in a quart-size bowl. Pour the milk over, stirring gently to mix. Cover and refrigerate overnight. In the morning, the chia seeds will have absorbed most of the almond milk and the mixture will have a thick, pudding-like consistency.

Take the kraut out of the jar with a clean fork, letting any extra brine drain back into it. Finely mince the kraut and stir it into the chia seed mixture, along with the pecans and coconut. Season to taste with salt. If you want a slightly thinner porridge, serve it with additional almond milk.

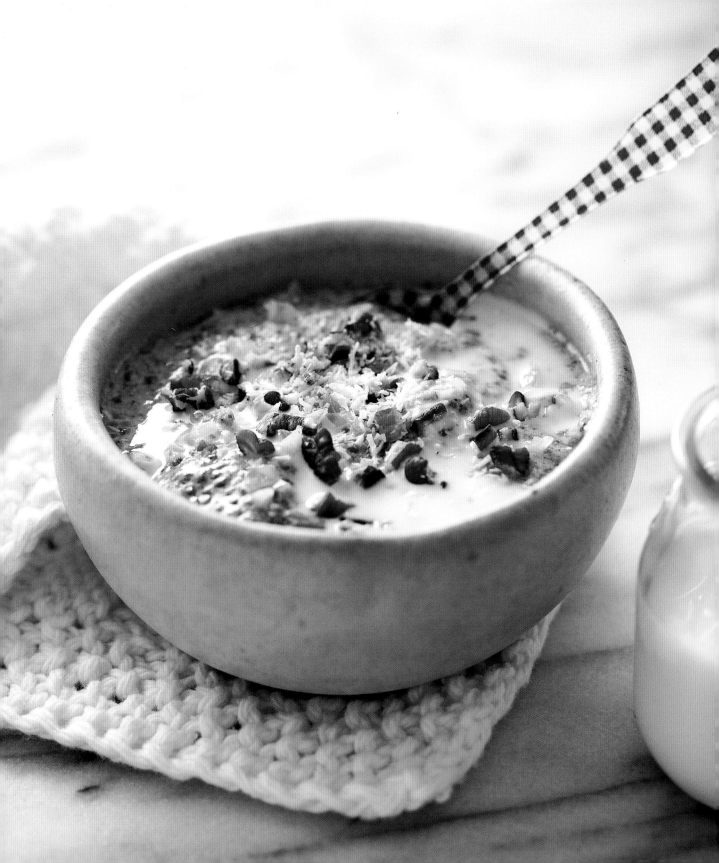

Kraut over Kitchari

Especially beneficial to those with compromised digestion, kitchari *(or khichdi) is a staple of ayurvedic cooking that traditionally includes split mung beans and rice. Common in many cultures around the world,* kitchari *is a comfort food, but it's also used frequently for detox cleansing since it is very easy to digest.*

Teri Adolfo, a Seattle based practitioner of ayurveda and acupuncture, shared one of her cleansing kitchari recipes with us. Here we use lentils instead of the traditional split mung beans so we have a more textured dish, but experiment with both to see what you like best. Also, quinoa or amaranth can be evenly substituted for some of the rice. Beets impart a gorgeous ruby hue and earthy sweetness, but don't hesitate to try fresh cut green beans, cubed yams, cut-up broccoli, or any vegetable that seems like a good fit to you.

One of the best parts about this recipe is the combination of garnishes that provide all the tastes—sweet, salty, sour, pungent, bitter, and astringent—that are essential to a traditional ayurvedic meal. The toppings really make this dish sparkle with the kraut adding that polishing touch on top. We like to think of this as a savory breakfast porridge, however, we like to eat leftovers for lunch or dinner.

Makes 6 to 8 servings

2 cups brown basmati rice

1 cup brown or green lentils

2 tablespoons coconut oil or ghee

1 teaspoon cumin seeds

1 teaspoon fennel seeds

1 teaspoon mustard seeds

2 cloves garlic, crushed and chopped

2 teaspoons coriander seeds

2 teaspoons minced fresh ginger

1 teaspoon ground turmeric

6½ cups water or stock (vegetable or chicken)

1 teaspoon salt

1 to 2 cups finely diced vegetables

In a small bowl, cover the rice with water and soak anywhere from 1 hour to overnight. (The longer you soak it, the more digestible it will be.) In a fine-mesh strainer, rinse the rice and lentils together until the water runs clear, drain, and set aside.

Melt the coconut oil in a medium pot over medium heat. Crush the cumin and fennel, then add the mustard seeds and sauté, stirring constantly, until the mustard seeds pop and the spices release their fragrance, about 1 minute. Add the garlic and sauté for 1 minute more.

Add the rice and lentils, and sauté for 2 more minutes, stirring to mix in the spices. Crush the coriander, then add the ginger and turmeric and sauté for 1 minute.

Add the water, salt, and vegetables, and bring the water to a boil. Reduce the heat to low, cover, and simmer until the liquid has been absorbed, about 35 to 45 minutes. (After 30 minutes, check to make sure the mixture isn't sticking; if it is, you may need to add more a tablespoon or two of water and continue cooking.) Remove the pot from the heat, and let cool slightly.

While the *kitchari* is cooking, take the kraut out of the jar with a clean fork, letting any extra brine drain back into it. Put the kraut in a blender and whirl it until it's the consistency of applesauce. Or mince it with a knife.

When you're ready to serve, portion the *kitchari* evenly into bowls and top with an equal amount of all the garnishes. Or let people serve themselves, both *kitchari* and toppings.

TOPPINGS:

1 cup Classic Kraut (page 29) or Caraway Kraut (page 41)

Lime wedges

Minced fresh ginger

Coconut oil

Unsweetened dried coconut flakes

Chopped fresh cilantro

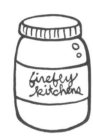

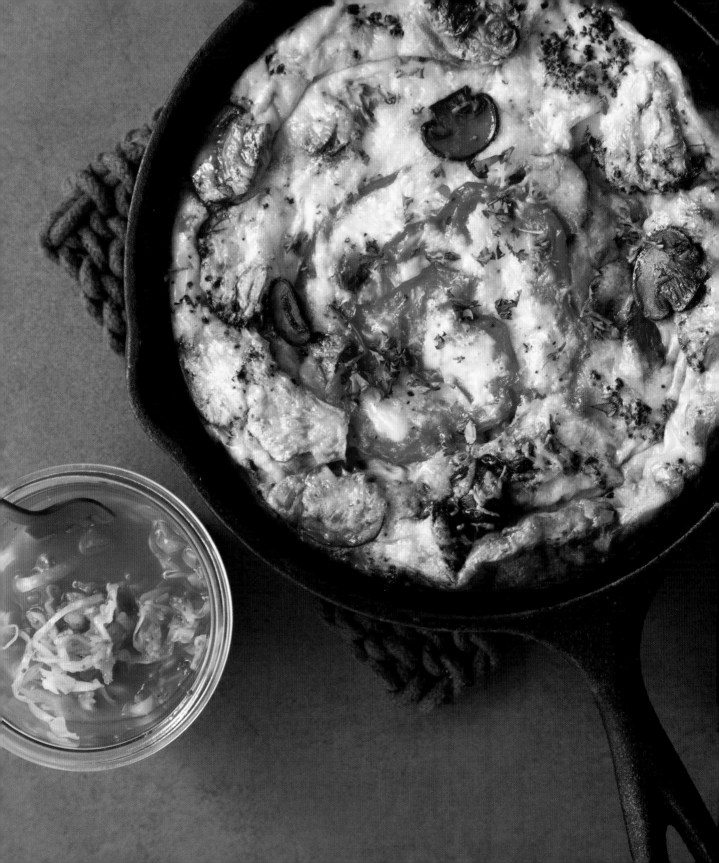

Not Your Mama's Frittata

Frittatas are a great way to get ample protein and a full serving of vegetables in your morning meal, and leftovers are perfect to pack for lunch. Play around with the ingredients depending on the season and make this dish your own. Some combos we love are: broccoli, ham, and Gruyère; tomato, basil, and mozzarella; chanterelle mushrooms, sage, and bacon; peas, prosciutto, and rosemary; potato and leek.

Preheat the oven to 375 degrees F.

Whisk the eggs, half-and-half, and salt in a medium bowl until the eggs are light and thoroughly blended. Set aside.

Melt the butter in a large ovenproof skillet—we love cast iron—over medium heat. Add the onions and sauté until they're translucent, about 10 minutes. Add the mushrooms and sauté until they're soft, another 4 to 5 minutes. Add the broccoli, bell pepper, salt, and pepper and sauté for another 2 to 3 minutes. Remove the skillet from the heat and stir in the parsley.

Spread this mixture evenly in the pan if you've used an ovenproof skillet. (You can also mix the veggies into the eggs and put them all into a greased 9-inch round, ovenproof baking dish or pie pan.)

Pour the whisked eggs over the vegetables. Sprinkle the Parmesan on top and bake until the eggs in the center don't jiggle (they'll be fairly solid to the touch) when you move the skillet, 25 to 30 minutes. Remove the frittata from the oven and let it cool for a few minutes.

While the frittata is baking, take the kimchi out of the jar with a clean fork, letting any extra brine drain back into it. Roughly chop the kimchi.

Serve the frittata right from the pan you baked it in. Cut it into wedges, top each wedge with a couple of tablespoons of kimchi, and serve immediately.

Makes 4 to 6 servings

8 large organic eggs

¼ cup half-and-half or milk of your choice

1 teaspoon salt

3 tablespoons butter or coconut oil

1 small yellow onion, diced

4 medium mushrooms, sliced

1 cup chopped broccoli florets

½ medium red bell pepper, chopped

1 teaspoon salt

½ teaspoon freshly ground black pepper

¼ cup chopped fresh parsley or basil

½ cup grated Parmesan cheese (about 2 ounces)

1 cup Firefly Kimchi (page 53)

Latkes with Crème Fraîche Kraut Sauce

Potato latkes, simple pancakes of grated potatoes, have a long history in both Europe and the Middle East. On their own, they can turn a breakfast routine into something special. For a protein boost, you can top them with a poached or fried egg, or they're particularly divine if you dollop them with Smoked Salmon Mousse (page 96) before you drizzle on the crème fraîche kraut sauce.

Although this recipe calls for Caraway Kraut, it pairs well with any ferment. Get creative by substituting sweet potatoes, yams, or carrots for half of the potatoes. If you're lucky enough to have leftover latkes, you can reheat them quickly in a skillet for an afternoon snack. A simple garnish is applesauce, with a little Classic Kraut (page 29) stirred in.

Makes 8 to 10 latkes

4 large russet potatoes (about 2 pounds)

2 tablespoons minced onion

2 tablespoons Caraway Kraut (page 41), chopped

3 tablespoons all-purpose or gluten-free flour

2 organic eggs, whisked until well blended

1½ teaspoons salt

½ teaspoon freshly ground black pepper

2 to 3 tablespoons coconut oil, peanut oil, or butter, for frying

Peel the potatoes if you want. (We use organic potatoes, so we usually leave the skin on.) Grate them using a handheld grater or a food processor's grater attachment. Immediately drop the grated potatoes into a large bowl of cold water and soak them for 2 minutes. Drain the potatoes thoroughly. Roll them up in a clean dish towel and twist the towel to squeeze out as much moisture as possible. Unwrap the potatoes, and put them in a medium bowl. Add the onion, kraut, and flour, and mix until evenly incorporated. Add the eggs, salt, and pepper, and mix well.

For each latke, scoop up about ⅓ cup of the mixture and shape it into a small patty. The latkes cook best when they're about ½ inch thick.

Heat the oil in a large fry or sauté pan over medium heat. Drop a small dollop of the batter into the pan to test the oil temperature; if the temperature is right, the batter should sizzle immediately. (Making sure the oil is hot enough will help the latkes brown evenly and absorb less oil.)

When the oil is hot, drop 3 or 4 latkes into the pan at a time, frying until golden brown, 3 to 4 minutes. Flip and repeat on the other side. Repeat this process until you've cooked all the latkes, adding more oil to the pan if needed. Put the cooked latkes on a wire rack or plate lined with paper towels to drain any excess oil. You can keep them warm in a 200-degree F oven until you're ready to serve them.

To make the sauce, combine all the ingredients except the salt and pepper in a small bowl. Season to taste with salt and pepper. Chill until ready to serve.

To serve, put 2 or 3 latkes on each plate. Dollop 1 or 2 tablespoons of sauce on top, and garnish with a sprig of parsley.

FOR THE SAUCE:

¼ cup Caraway Kraut (page 41), roughly chopped

½ cup crème fraîche, sour cream, or plain Greek yogurt

Salt and freshly ground black pepper

Parsley sprigs, for garnish

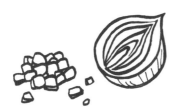

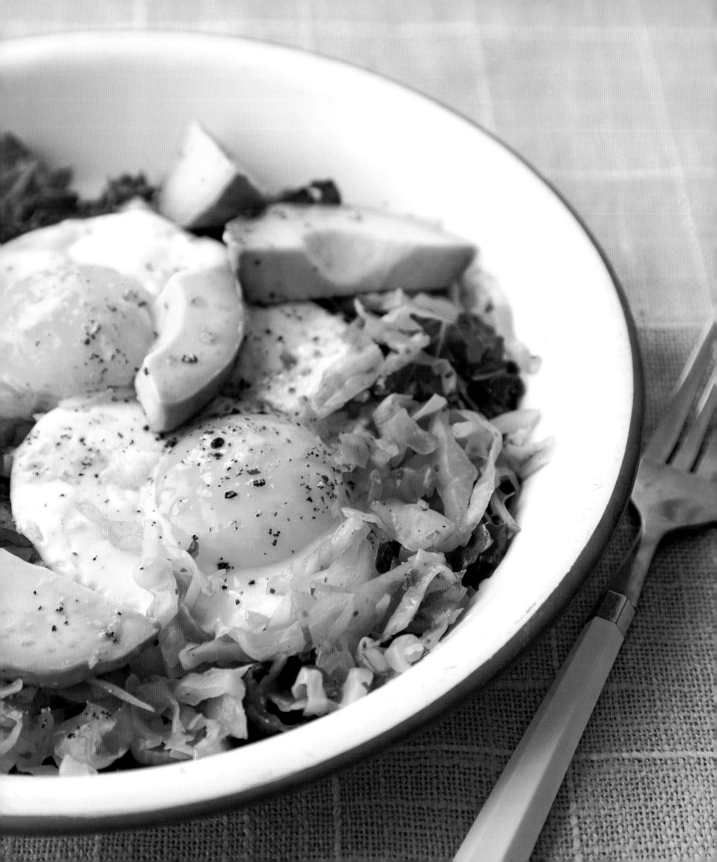

Kimchi Kick-Start Breakfast

This breakfast combo of nutrient- and fiber-rich leafy greens, protein, healthy fats, and, of course, probiotics and digestive enzymes jump-starts your metabolism and energy production while keeping your blood sugar stable. Our secret to cooking over-easy eggs is to add a splash of water—or better yet, kimchi brine—to the pan. Cover the pan and cook the eggs for about two minutes, or until they're done the way you like them. No messy flipping involved, and your eggs will come out just right!

Melt 4 tablespoons of the butter in a large skillet over medium heat. Add the onions and sauté until they're translucent, about 10 minutes.

While the onions cook, cut or tear the kale leaves from the thick stalks, discarding the stalks (if you're using Swiss chard, you can save them for another use). Slice the kale leaves into ¼-inch strips (you should have about 4 cups). Add the kale to the skillet with the onions, and cook until it's wilted and tender, an additional 6 to 8 minutes. Season the kale mixture to taste with salt and pepper, and divide it between two to four plates.

Fry the eggs in the remaining 2 teaspoons of butter for about 2 minutes, or until they're done the way you like them.

To serve, place egg or eggs on top of each mound of kale and arrange the avocado slices right on top. Take the kimchi out of the jar with a clean fork, letting any extra brine drain back into it. Top each egg with ¼ cup kimchi. Drizzle 1 to 2 teaspoons of kimchi brine over the top of each dish to add a splash of flavor. Serve warm.

Makes 2 to 4 servings

4 tablespoons plus 2 teaspoons butter or coconut oil, divided

1 small yellow onion, sliced into thin half moons

¾ pound kale or Swiss chard

Salt and freshly ground black pepper

4 organic eggs

1 large avocado, halved, pitted, peeled, and cut into ¼-inch wedges

1 cup Firefly Kimchi (page 53)

2 to 4 teaspoons brine (optional)

Breakfast Burritos 3 Krauty Ways

Breakfast burritos are one of the easiest, most protein-packed breakfasts to make on the fly, and a great way to use up leftovers. Almost any veggie or meat will scramble up well with a base of eggs and onions. Get creative with what you have on hand and experiment with other combinations.

Serve the eggs in the traditional burrito style, wrapped in a warm flour tortilla, or try them taco-style in warm corn tortillas. For a tortilla-free version, pair the eggs with Latkes with Crème Fraîche Kraut Sauce (page 86) or a sautéed green, such as spinach.

Makes 4 servings

1 tablespoon butter

½ large yellow onion, minced

½ teaspoon salt

6 organic eggs, beaten

4 medium flour or corn tortillas

1 cup Firefly Kimchi (page 53), or your favorite kraut

The Basic

Melt the butter in a large sauté pan over medium-high heat. Add the onions and salt, and cook until the onions are translucent, about 10 minutes. Add the eggs and cook, stirring frequently, until scrambled, about 4 minutes. Remove the pan from the heat as soon as they're done.

While the eggs are cooking, warm the tortillas in a separate skillet over medium heat.

To serve, scoop ¼ of the egg mixture into each warm tortilla. Top the eggs with kraut then roll up the tortilla burrito-style and serve immediately.

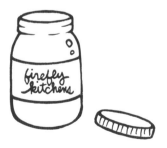

Variations

JALAPEÑO, BACON, AND CORTIDO KRAUT: After the onions have cooked for 5 minutes, add 1 to 2 tablespoons minced jalapeño and 6 strips diced bacon. Cook until the bacon gets brown and slightly crispy, another 5 minutes or so.

SAUSAGE, GREENS, AND CARAWAY KRAUT: After the onions have cooked for 5 minutes, add ¼ pound Italian or breakfast sausages, cut into ¼-inch pieces. Sauté until the sausage is fully cooked, another 5 minutes or so. Add the eggs and cook, stirring frequently, for 2 minutes. Add 2 cups kale, Swiss chard, or collard greens, stemmed and cut into thin ribbons, and cook for another 2 minutes, or until the eggs are scrambled and the kale is slightly wilted.

VEGGIE AND EMERALD CITY KRAUT: After the onions have cooked for 5 minutes, add 1 cup (2 small) finely diced red or golden potatoes. Sauté until the potatoes are soft and cooked through, another 8 to 10 minutes. Add 2 medium mushrooms and ¼ red bell pepper, diced, and cook until the moisture from the mushrooms has evaporated, 4 to 6 minutes.

Chapter 6:
Quick Bites

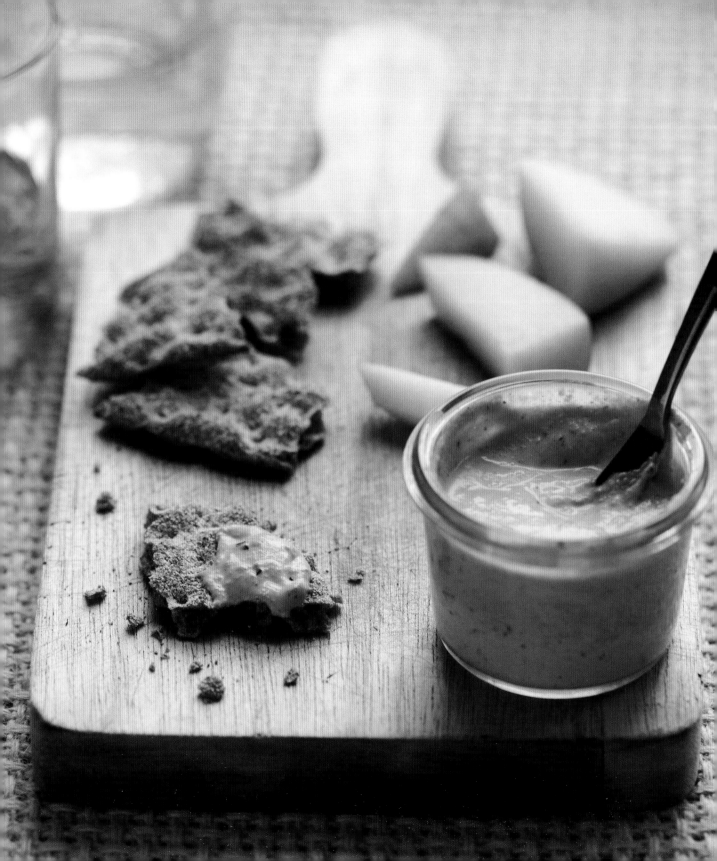

Firefly Kimcheese

This is by far our most sought-after recipe and the one we made to celebrate winning our first Good Food Award. We suggest making a double batch because you'll want to eat it with everything!

Our original was the Make It Quick & Simple recipe, but over time it has turned into the richer, creamier version below. It's always the biggest hit at our Fermented Happy Hour, where we serve it as a delectable dip with veggies and crackers.

Experiment! Add a bit of extra kimchi brine to thin it and stir it into pasta, or add a bit more cheese to make a thicker spread for sandwiches or wraps. It's also great slathered on any burger.

Take the kimchi out of the jar with a clean fork, letting any extra brine drain back into it. Whirl the kimchi in a food processor for 1 minute. Add the cream cheese, goat cheese, and garlic, and blend for another 30 seconds. Add the parsley and hot sauce, and pulse a few more times until the cheese is smooth. If it's too thick for your liking, add a splash of brine or oil. Season to taste with salt and pepper. Serve chilled.

Make It Quick & Simple

Whirl ¾ cup Firefly Kimchi and 8 ounces cream cheese in a food processor.

Makes about 2 cups

¾ cup Firefly Kimchi (page 53)

8 ounces cream cheese

¼ cup goat cheese (1 ounce) (optional)

1 clove garlic, crushed

1 tablespoon chopped fresh parsley

1 teaspoon Sriracha, or your favorite hot sauce

Brine or extra-virgin olive oil, for thinning

Salt and freshly ground black pepper

Smoked Salmon Mousse

This is such a decadent treat that, if you make it for guests, you may want to hide it in the back of the fridge so you don't devour it before they arrive! Any style of smoked salmon will work well in this recipe, though we typically use softer varieties like lox.

A great everyday snack with crackers and veggies, this mousse makes an especially luscious topping for a risotto or pasta. You can also spoon it into tart shells for an elegant (but easy) start to a special meal.

Makes about 2 cups

½ cup Classic Kraut (page 29)

½ pound smoked salmon

8 ounces cream cheese

⅓ cup mayonnaise, plain yogurt, or sour cream

1 green onion, thinly sliced, including the green tops

2 tablespoons chopped fresh parsley

Splash of Tabasco

Pinch of dried dill

Take the kraut out of the jar with a clean fork, letting any extra brine drain back into it. Blend the kraut and smoked salmon in a food processor for about 30 seconds. Add the cream cheese and blend for 1 minute. Add the mayonnaise, green onion, parsley, Tabasco, and dill, and blend for 1 minute, or a bit longer for a lighter, fluffier mousse.

Make It Quick & Simple

Emerald City Kraut adds a touch of dill and kale to this simple mousse. Blend 8 ounces cream cheese, ½ pound smoked salmon, and ½ cup Emerald City Kraut (page 49) until you get the texture you want.

Olive Bean Tapenade

This white bean dip's bright flavor is enjoyable on just about every type of cracker or bread it meets and any other edible vehicle you have around, such as carrots, endive, or celery. In fact, when we have some in the lunch fridge at Firefly Kitchens, we've been known to eat it right out of the jar we keep it in.

Try adding a couple of tablespoons of tahini for a richer tapenade. To achieve a completely smooth texture for a sandwich spread or a dip, simply whirl all the ingredients in a food processor. Or leave it chunky to spread on bread or crackers.

Take the kraut out of the jar with a clean fork, letting any extra brine drain back into it. Roughly chop the kraut and combine it with the beans and olives in a medium bowl. Add the lemon zest, red pepper flakes, lemon juice, parsley, basil, and oil, and toss to incorporate. Use the back of a fork or a potato masher to smash the beans until the mixture is the consistency you want. Season to taste with salt and pepper. Chill until ready to serve.

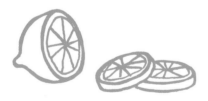

Makes about 5 cups

½ cup Classic Kraut (page 29)

1½ cups cooked white beans, or 1 (15-ounce) can, drained and rinsed (see Legumes, page 215, for cooking instructions)

¾ cup chopped, pitted Kalamata olives

Zest of ½ lemon (about 1 teaspoon)

½ teaspoon red pepper flakes

1 tablespoon freshly squeezed lemon juice

2 tablespoons finely chopped fresh parsley

2 tablespoons finely chopped fresh basil (optional)

1 tablespoon extra-virgin olive oil

Salt and freshly ground black pepper

Ruby Tuna Pâté

Talk about nirvana on the palate—Richard's pâté recipe is complex and rich, yet simple to make. The vibrant red of the beets brightens the pâté and adds a healthy dose of antioxidants. Serve it with crackers or scooped onto some cucumber rounds as an appetizer (it's a bit more spreadable than a traditional pâté). Add a squeeze of lemon, a splash of brandy, or minced herbs for an extra kick. You might even add extra kraut and turn it into a zesty dip.

Makes about 2 cups

½ cup pecans

2 teaspoons butter or
  coconut oil

½ yellow onion, diced

3 medium mushrooms, sliced

¾ cup Ruby Red Kraut
  (page 43)

2 tablespoons shredded organic
  raw beets

1 (5-ounce) can wild-caught
  tuna, drained

⅓ cup grated Parmesan cheese
  (about 1.5 ounces)

2 tablespoons chopped fresh
  parsley

Salt and freshly ground black
  pepper

Toast the pecans in a small skillet over low heat. Stir constantly (they burn easily) until they're browned and fragrant, 5 to 8 minutes. Set aside.

Melt the butter in a skillet over medium heat. Add the onions and sauté until they're translucent, about 10 minutes. Add the mushrooms and sauté until they're lightly browned, another 5 to 8 minutes. Set aside.

Take the kraut out of the jar with a clean fork, letting any extra brine drain back into it.

Squeeze out any extra brine before adding kraut into a food processor with the beets and tuna and blending for about 1 minute.

Scrape down the sides of the bowl. Add the pecans, onion mixture, Parmesan, and parsley. Blend until you have a creamy texture, about 1 to 2 minutes. Season to taste with salt and pepper.

Limacado Dip

Whoever said lima beans don't taste good is wrong, but you can substitute white beans if you're not convinced. This lightly spiced dip makes a delicious substitute for traditional guacamole and serves as a flavorful sauce on grilled meat or in tacos. It's fun to ask guests to try to guess the ingredients!

Take the kraut out of the jar with a clean fork, letting any extra brine drain back into it. Put the kraut, garlic, red onion, and jalapeño in a food processor, and pulse until roughly chopped, about 1 minute. Add the lima beans and pulse for another 30 seconds. Add the avocado, lemon juice, cilantro, cumin, and salt, and pulse until smooth. Season to taste with pepper and hot sauce, adding additional salt, if desired.

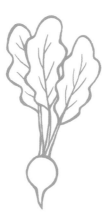

Makes about 2 cups

½ cup Cortido Kraut (page 47)

2 to 3 cloves garlic

¼ cup diced red onion

½ medium jalapeño, with seeds, chopped

1½ cups cooked lima beans, or 1 (15-ounce) can, drained and rinsed (see Legumes, page 215, for cooking instructions)

1 ripe avocado, halved, pitted, and peeled

1 tablespoon freshly squeezed lemon juice

3 tablespoons chopped fresh cilantro

¼ teaspoon ground cumin

½ teaspoon salt

Freshly ground black pepper

Your favorite hot sauce

Firefly Lentil Pâté

Everyone who tries this recipe says, "I could eat this every day!" In fact, this pâté is as nutritious as it is appetizing, so why not always keep a batch in your refrigerator?

Loaded with protein, lentils are a cholesterol-lowering legume and rich in B vitamins. Red, green, brown, or French lentils all work beautifully in this recipe.

This is more of a spreading than a slicing pâté, and you can also make it into a dip by adding a splash of brine or olive oil to thin it out. For an elegant starter, add a couple of drops of truffle oil or a pinch of truffle salt along with the lentils and parsley.

Makes 4 cups

½ cup pecans

1 cup Firefly Kimchi (page 53)

½ cup Caramelized Onions (recipe follows)

2 cups cooked lentils (see Legumes, page 215, for cooking instructions)

3 tablespoons roughly chopped fresh parsley

1 clove garlic, crushed

3 tablespoons softened butter (optional)

1 teaspoon brandy (optional)

Salt and freshly ground black pepper

Toast the pecans in a small skillet over low heat. Stir constantly (they burn easily) until they're browned and fragrant, 5 to 8 minutes.

Take the kimchi out of the jar with a clean fork, letting any extra brine drain back into it. Whirl it in a food processor until it's the consistency of applesauce. Scrape down the bowl, add the pecans and onions, and blend for another 30 seconds. Add the lentils, parsley, garlic, butter, and brandy, and pulse until well mixed. Season to taste with salt and pepper.

NOTE: If you don't have time to caramelize the onions (it takes upwards of half an hour), you can just thinly slice half a large onion (about 1½ cups), then sauté the slices in a tablespoon of olive oil with a pinch of brown sugar (to re-create the sweetness of caramelized onions) until the onions are translucent, about 10 minutes.

Caramelized Onions

Caramelized onions can truly transform a meal, so try making a batch to have them on hand during the week to top off salad, spread on a sandwich, or use as a base for a quick veggie sauté. The longer you cook them, the more their sugars will release, so be patient and let them work their magic. Keep these sweet onions in the fridge for about five days; they also freeze well in ice cube trays or small containers.

Heat a large, heavy sauté pan over medium-high heat and add the butter and oil. When the oil just begins to sizzle, add the onions and toss to coat them. Reduce the heat to medium-low, sprinkle in the salt, and toss once more. Cook, stirring only occasionally, for at least 15 minutes or up to an hour. If the onions start to stick, add a touch of water, broth, or wine to the bottom of the pan and scrape to release the flavorful browned bits that also add color to the onions.

2 tablespoons butter

2 tablespoons extra-virgin olive oil

4 large onions, halved and sliced into thin half moons (about 8 cups)

2 teaspoons salt

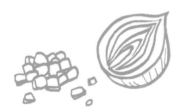

Strawberry Yin Yang Salsa

This salsa is best made with the freshest, ripest strawberries you can find. Eat it right away so the berries don't get mushy and you don't lose the delicate intensity of their flavor. (If you missed the strawberry season, perfectly ripe blueberries or stone fruit, such as peaches and nectarines, make a great substitute.) Their vibrant sweet flavor infuses the rest of the ingredients, balancing the sourness of the carrots and lime, to create a refreshing topping for any fish or grain. Add an extra tablespoon of olive oil and balsamic vinegar and toss this salsa with any leafy greens salad to turn an ordinary salad into something special.

Makes about 2 cups

¾ cup Yin Yang Carrots
(page 55)

2 cups sliced fresh strawberries
(about 1 pint)

1 tablespoon apple cider
vinegar

6 to 8 basil leaves, thinly sliced

2 green onions, thinly sliced,
including the green tops

Juice of ½ medium lime (about
1 tablespoon)

1 tablespoon extra-virgin olive
oil

¼ teaspoon salt

Take the carrots out of the jar with a clean fork, letting any extra brine drain back into it. Gently mix the carrots and strawberries in a medium bowl. Add the remaining ingredients, and toss lightly so you don't smash the berries. Serve right away.

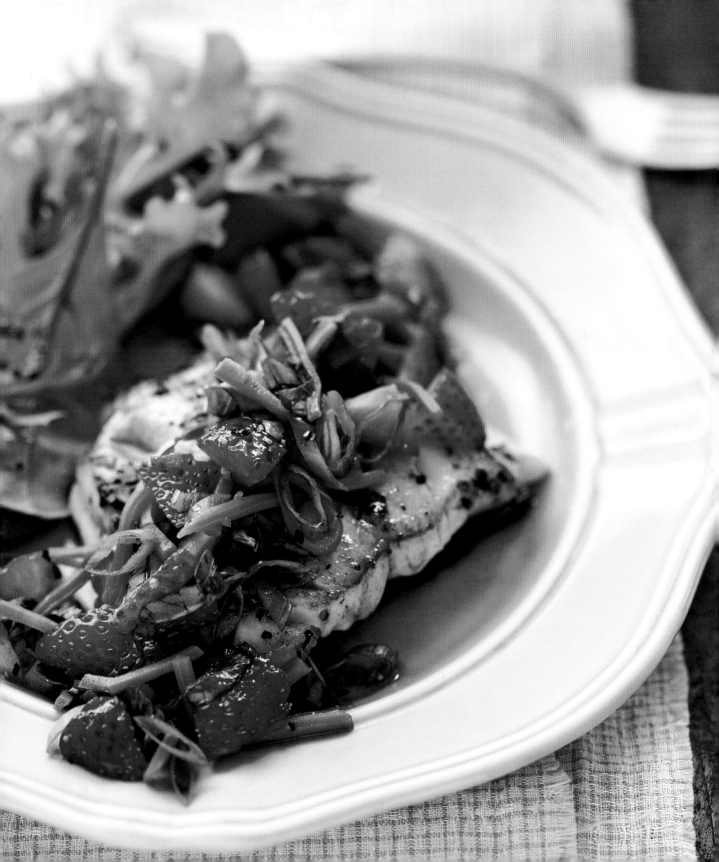

Sun-Dried Tomato Tapenade

This Mediterranean-inspired tapenade gives you a tomato hit when there are no vine-ripe tomatoes to be found. Our favorite way to serve it is with a soft, creamy cheese and crisp whole-grain crackers as a versatile snack or appetizer. You can blend in some cream cheese for a richer dip. Or get creative with toasted pine nuts, walnuts, capers, Kalamata olives, or fresh basil. Use it to spark up a pasta salad, or find it featured in the Sun-Dried Tomato Linguine (page 192).

Makes about 2 cups

1 cup Ruby Red Kraut (page 43)

½ cup oil-packed sun-dried tomatoes, drained

2 cloves garlic, crushed

2 tablespoons minced fresh parsley

2 tablespoons extra-virgin olive oil

1 teaspoon Dijon mustard

2 anchovies (optional)

Salt and freshly ground black pepper

Take the kraut out of the jar with a clean fork, letting any extra brine drain back into it. Put the kraut and sun-dried tomatoes in a food processor and blend for 1 minute. Add the garlic, parsley, oil, mustard, and anchovies, and whirl until smooth. Season to taste with salt and pepper.

PB Chi Spread

We created this spread one day while we were dreaming about the peanut sauce in Mollie Katzen's tofu and broccoli dish from The Enchanted Broccoli Forest, *which has been a favorite of Julie's for over twenty-five years. Molly and her timeless classic vegetarian cookbooks are a repeated source of inspiration and ideas for Firefly Kitchens, reminding us that there is never an end to creativity and innovation when it comes to cooking and sharing delicious food with others.*

Creamy and zesty, this spread also makes a luscious sauce on top of just about anything— chicken, broccoli, rice, or tofu. Or use it as a dip for cucumber slices or celery sticks (you get the idea!). We love it so much, we even created a dish, Chicken Satay with Rice Noodles (page 173), that features it.

In a food processor, whirl all of the ingredients except the salt and pepper until smooth. Add a splash of water or brine if you want it thinner. Season to taste with salt and pepper.

Make It Quick & Simple

If you're in a rush, whirl 1 cup peanut butter and 1 cup Firefly Kimchi in a food processor until smooth. Add as much water or brine as you need to thin it to the consistency you want.

Makes about 3 cups

1 cup Firefly Kimchi (page 53)

1 cup organic peanut butter

½ cup warm water

1 tablespoon apple cider vinegar

1 tablespoon tamari

1 tablespoon molasses

2 cloves garlic, minced

1 to 2 green onions, thinly sliced, including the green tops

1 teaspoon minced fresh ginger

Pinch of cayenne pepper

Salt and freshly ground black pepper

Edamame Hummus

Edamame, common to Japanese and Chinese cooking, are immature soybeans, usually served in the pod. These beans are incredibly high in protein, fiber, and estrogen-mimicking isoflavones.

This hummus, lighter and fluffier than that made from chickpeas, has a surprisingly brilliant-green color—perfect for a Saint Patrick's Day treat. It's a dip for chips and veggies, but it's also great as a spread on sandwiches and wraps. Or you can thin it with olive oil and use it as a dressing for salads and slaws.

For a more herbal, pesto-like flavor, use the basil and parsley (or any other herbs you like), as well as the green onions. Omit the herbs for a more classic and subtle hummus spiked with the heat of wasabi—of course, the more wasabi you add, the sharper the flavor.

Makes about 3 cups

2 cups frozen shelled edamame

2 to 3 cloves garlic, minced

⅓ cup extra-virgin olive oil

¼ cup tahini

1 to 3 teaspoons wasabi paste, or ½ teaspoon wasabi powder

½ teaspoon lemon zest

Juice of 1 small lemon (about 2 tablespoons)

1½ teaspoons salt

½ teaspoon freshly ground black pepper

2 tablespoons chopped fresh basil (optional)

1 tablespoon chopped fresh parsley (optional)

1 tablespoon chopped green onion (optional)

⅓ cup Classic Kraut (page 29)

1 cup cooked or canned chickpeas, drained (see Legumes, page 215, for cooking instructions)

Cook the edamame in lightly salted water for 5 minutes. Drain and set aside.

Put the garlic, oil, tahini, wasabi, lemon zest, lemon juice, salt, pepper, basil, parsley, and green onion in a blender or food processor, and whirl until smooth.

Take the kraut out of the jar with a clean fork, letting any extra brine drain back into it. Add the kraut to the tahini-herb mixture, along with the edamame and chickpeas, and whirl until smooth—the longer you whirl it, the smoother it will be. (You may need to thin it with additional oil or brine to keep things moving in the blender.)

> **NOTE:** If you like a chunkier hummus, don't whirl the edamame, chickpeas, and kraut; instead just pulse until you like what you see.

Creamy Kraut Salsa

One of our New York friends, Sharon Parsons, gave us the thumbs-up to use this recipe in our book. Of course we had to tweak it and sneak in some kraut.

A bright combo of salsa and guacamole with an extra kick and crunch, this dish will steal the show. Creamy-smooth avocado, peppery heat, zesty herbs, fresh tomatoes, and crunchy cucumbers unite to create a dip that satisfies both salsa and guacamole lovers alike. Mango, stone fruit, berries, pineapple, and tomatillos, as well as other ferments such as Ruby Red Kraut (page 43) and Cortido Kraut (page 47), make great additions. And never hesitate to toss in more kraut.

Take the kraut out of the jar with a clean fork, letting any extra brine drain back into it. Roughly chop the kraut and mix it with the remaining ingredients in a medium bowl. Season to taste with additional salt and pepper if needed. Serve immediately.

FREEZING FRESH HERBS

If you have an excess of fresh herbs, such as parsley, cilantro, or basil, simply chop them up and freeze them in an ice cube tray with water to cover. (The water keeps the herbs from freezer burns.) Store the herby cubes in a ziplock bag and thaw as needed; they make a great addition to soups, sauces, or stir-fries.

Makes 4 cups

½ cup Classic Kraut (page 29)

3 medium tomatoes, seeded and diced

2 medium avocados, halved, pitted, peeled, and diced

1 medium cucumber, peeled, seeded, and finely diced

1 stalk celery, finely diced

1 medium jalapeño, seeded and minced

2 tablespoons finely chopped fresh basil

¼ cup finely chopped fresh cilantro

Juice of 1 medium lemon (about 3 tablespoons)

Juice of 1 medium lime (about 2 tablespoon)

2 tablespoons extra-virgin olive oil

1 to 2 tablespoons apple cider vinegar or white balsamic vinegar

1 teaspoon salt

½ teaspoon freshly ground black pepper

Mango Avocado Salsa

Sweet mango, creamy avocado, and zippy citrus and kraut make a great combination in this fresh summer salsa. Like any salsa, this is good with crackers and chips, but it's also a refreshing counterpoint to a piece of grilled fish or tofu (or any grilled meat). It also makes a sweet addition to salads and wraps—a great way to use up any leftovers.

The color of the Ruby Red Kraut is beautiful in the mix, but Classic Kraut (page 29) will work well too. To kick the spice up a notch, use the jalapeño seeds. Ripe papaya makes a perfect substitute for mango in this salsa—so perfect that you should choose whichever fruit is ripest.

Makes about 2 cups

¾ cup Ruby Red Kraut (page 43)

1 large avocado, halved, pitted, peeled, and diced

1 medium mango, peeled, pitted, and diced

¼ cup finely diced red onion

1 small jalapeño, seeded and minced (about 1 tablespoon)

1 tablespoon apple cider vinegar

Juice of 1 medium lime (about 2 tablespoons)

1 tablespoon extra-virgin olive oil

Salt

Take the kraut out of the jar with a clean fork, letting any extra brine drain back into it. Roughly chop the kraut, and mix it with all the remaining ingredients except the salt in a medium bowl. Season to taste with salt. Serve immediately or refrigerate for up to 1 hour before serving.

Chapter 7:
Salads for Noon & Night

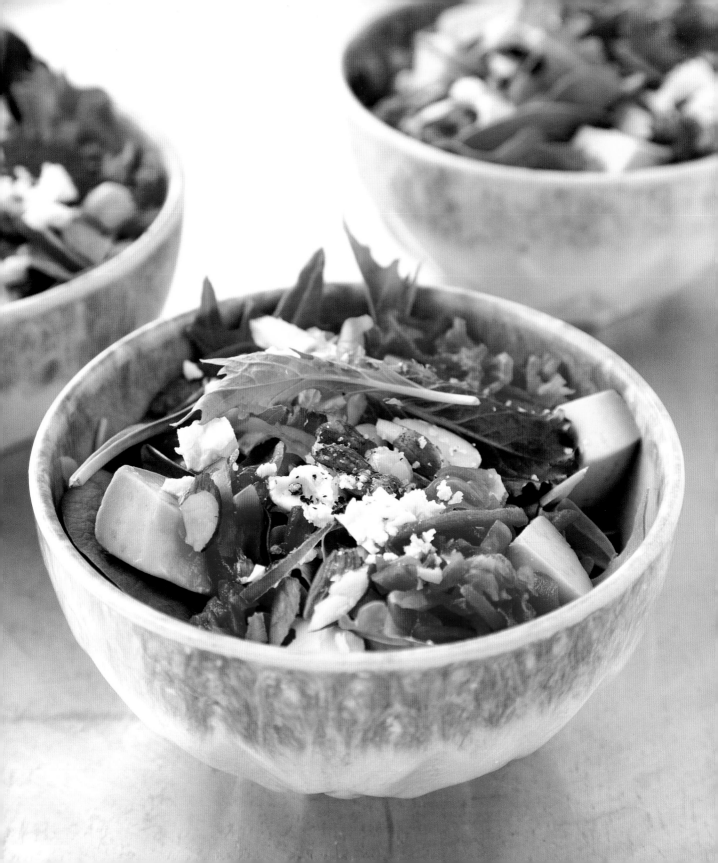

PowerKraut Salad

When Firefly first started selling products at Seattle farmers' markets, our customers would always ask us for ideas about how to use them. We were trying to get people to think out of the box when it comes to kraut. Kraut isn't just a topping for sausage, we would tell them. Try it in salads, with roasted vegetables, or blended into hummus.

Eventually we printed up recipe cards to share; this salad was Firefly's first official recipe. Since then we've added a few things, and the result is a hearty, nourishing bowl of greens, veggies, legumes, nuts, and seeds that make a satisfying meal. We especially love it for lunch because it fills you up without weighing you down. Ruby Red Kraut is our first pick for this salad because of its vibrant color, but Classic Kraut (page 29) and Emerald City Kraut (page 49) are delicious too.

Toast the pumpkin seeds in a small skillet over low heat. Stir constantly (they burn easily) until they're golden brown, 5 to 7 minutes. Set them aside to cool.

Take the kraut out of the jar with a clean fork, letting any extra brine drain back into it. Roughly chop the kraut. Put the kraut with the pumpkin seeds in a large salad bowl, add the greens, avocado, onion, quinoa, and cheese, and toss to combine.

To make the dressing, whisk all the ingredients in a small bowl until smooth.

Pour the dressing over the salad and toss to evenly coat. Season to taste with salt and pepper, and serve immediately.

Makes 4 to 6 servings

½ cup raw pumpkin seeds or slivered almonds

1 cup Ruby Red Kraut (page 43)

6 cups slightly packed leafy greens (about 8 ounces)

1 large avocado, peeled, pitted, and diced

⅓ cup thinly sliced red onion

1 cup cooked quinoa (see Quinoa, page 216, for cooking instructions)

⅓ cup crumbled goat or feta cheese (about 1.5 ounces)

FOR THE DRESSING:

¼ cup apple cider vinegar

2 tablespoons extra-virgin olive oil

1 tablespoon freshly squeezed lemon or lime juice

2 teaspoons honey

Salt and freshly ground black pepper

Curried Carrot Quinoa Salad

This is a lunchtime favorite at Firefly Kitchens. Quinoa, with its high protein content, makes this a nourishing staple. Add mint or other seasonal herbs to tweak the salad's flavor, or toss in chickpeas, white beans, or sliced chicken or turkey to make a more substantial meal. This salad is a great one to make ahead because the longer it sits, the more its flavors develop, so it tastes even better the next day.

Makes 4 to 6 servings

FOR THE DRESSING:

1 tablespoon apple cider or rice wine vinegar

Juice of 1 medium lemon (about 3 tablespoons)

2 teaspoons curry powder

⅓ cup extra-virgin olive oil

¼ cup chopped fresh basil or parsley

¼ cup chopped fresh cilantro

1½ cups Yin Yang Carrots (page 55)

1 small red bell pepper, chopped

4 cups cooked quinoa (see Quinoa, page 216, for cooking instructions)

½ cup dried cranberries or cherries, chopped

½ cup pistachios, almonds, or cashews, chopped

Salt and freshly ground black pepper

To make the dressing, combine all the ingredients in a medium bowl. Let sit for 5 minutes while you make the salad.

Take the carrots out of the jar with a clean fork, letting any extra brine drain back into it. In a large bowl, toss the carrots with the bell pepper, quinoa, cranberries, and pistachios. Pour the dressing over the salad and toss to coat. Season to taste with salt and pepper. Serve right away or refrigerate for up to 2 days.

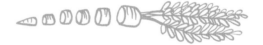

Emerald City Salad

This salad is one of our favorites in spring and early summer. Fresh strawberries from the garden or local farmers' market add a delicate sweetness that balances the flavorful kraut. If strawberries aren't in season, get the sweetness by substituting half an orange, thinly sliced. This salad is a wonderful accompaniment to any type of chicken or fish.

Take the kraut out of the jar with a clean fork, letting any extra brine drain back into it. Roughly chop the kraut. Put it in a large bowl, along with the remaining ingredients except the salt and pepper, and toss to combine. Refrigerate until ready to serve.

To make the dressing, start by crushing the coriander seeds using a mortar and pestle, a rolling pin, or a clean coffee grinder. Break the seeds down, but don't crush them to a powder. In a small bowl, whisk the crushed coriander together with all the remaining ingredients.

Just before serving, pour the vinaigrette over the salad and toss to coat. Season to taste with salt and pepper, and serve immediately.

Makes 4 to 6 servings

1 cup Emerald City Kraut (page 49)

1½ cups cooked or canned chickpeas (see Legumes, page 215, for cooking instructions)

4 cups lightly packed leafy greens (about 6 ounces)

1 cup thinly sliced strawberries (about ½ pint)

⅓ cup thinly sliced red onion (optional)

2 to 3 tablespoons crumbled goat cheese (optional)

Salt and freshly ground black pepper

FOR THE DRESSING:

1 teaspoon coriander seeds

Zest of 1 small orange (about 1 tablespoon)

2 tablespoons freshly squeezed orange juice

2 tablespoons champagne vinegar or other sweet vinegar

3 tablespoons extra-virgin olive oil

Krauty Kale Caesar

One of Firefly's first employees, Sarah Betts, shared this recipe with us—a "secret" recipe she doesn't give out to many. "This recipe is the reason people keep coming over to my house for dinner," she jokes. But in all honesty, it's one of the best Caesar dressings out there, with the kraut adding just the right amount of tang to brighten and lighten the creamy dressing.

Massaging the kale, as funny as it sounds, is important because it helps soften it, making the tough leaves easier to chew and digest. Croutons make a crunchy (and traditional) addition to this Caesar. Add chunks of roast chicken or grilled salmon, or chop up a hard-boiled egg or two, to make this a complete meal.

Makes 4 to 6 servings

2 large bunches kale (about 2 pounds)

FOR THE DRESSING:

2 tablespoons Dijon mustard

4 to 5 cloves garlic

¼ cup mayonnaise

¾ cup Classic Kraut (page 29)

1 tablespoon Worcestershire sauce

¼ cup extra-virgin olive oil

⅓ cup grated Parmesan cheese (about 1.5 ounces), plus additional for garnish

Juice of 2 small lemons (about ½ cup)

4 anchovies (optional)

Salt and freshly ground black pepper

Cut or tear the kale leaves from the thick stalks, discarding the stalks. Tear the leaves into small pieces and put them in a large bowl.

To make the dressing, whirl all the ingredients except the salt and pepper in a blender or food processor until smooth.

Pour the dressing over the kale. Using your hands, massage the dressing into the leaves until they start to soften, 2 to 3 minutes. (You can also accomplish this by tossing the salad vigorously with two wooden spoons.) Season to taste with salt and pepper, garnish with additional Parmesan, and serve immediately.

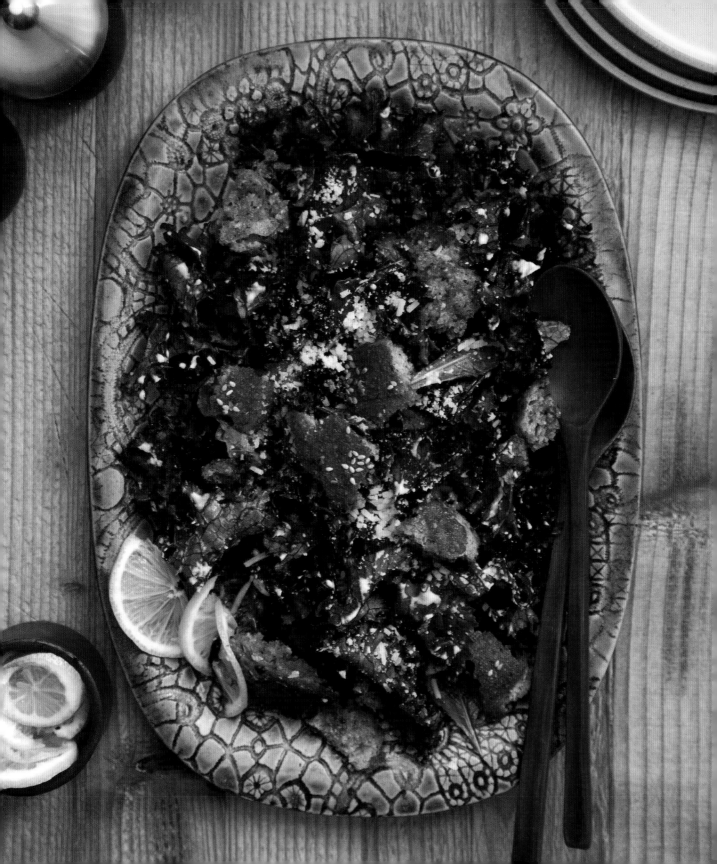

Greek Orzo Salad

This recipe feeds an army, or a bunch of hungry kids. It also makes great leftovers, so don't worry about finishing it all in one meal. Pack it up for lunch the following day or serve it over a bed of greens for a quick dinner the next night.

To make this salad an even more complete meal, add chunks of roasted eggplant or steamed green beans. Instead of Classic Kraut, try Ruby Red Kraut (page 43) or Caraway Kraut (page 41) for a richer, spicy flavor that complements the briny olives well.

Makes 6 to 8 servings

2 quarts water

2 teaspoons salt

1½ cups orzo pasta

1 cup Classic Kraut (page 29)

¾ cup crumbled feta cheese (about 3.5 ounces)

½ cup pitted Kalamata olives, roughly chopped

½ cup finely chopped red onion

½ cup finely chopped fresh parsley

1 large red bell pepper, cored, seeded, and chopped (about 1½ cups)

1½ cups halved cherry tomatoes

Salt and freshly ground black pepper

FOR THE DRESSING:

3 tablespoons extra-virgin olive oil

½ teaspoon dried basil, or 1 tablespoon chopped fresh basil

1 teaspoon Dijon mustard

1 teaspoon lemon zest

Juice of 1 small lemon (about 2 tablespoons)

2 tablespoons Classic Kraut (page 29)

1 teaspoon red wine vinegar

2 teaspoons Worcestershire sauce

Put the water and salt in a large pot, and bring it to a boil. Add the orzo and cook until it's tender yet firm to the bite, about 12 minutes. Drain the orzo and rinse it with cold water.

Take the kraut out of the jar with a clean fork, letting any extra brine drain back into it. Roughly chop the kraut. Put the orzo and kraut in a large bowl and toss with all the remaining ingredients except the salt and pepper.

To make the dressing, whirl all the dressing ingredients in a blender or food processor. Toss the orzo mixture with the dressing until thoroughly combined.

Season to taste with salt and pepper. Serve immediately or refrigerate for up to 1 day.

Green Bean Potato Salad

The classic potato salad never gets old, but it's fun to dress it up now and again. Green beans add great color and a satisfying crunch to the tender potatoes, while the earthy flavor of caraway lingers in each bite, creating a deeper and more interesting taste.

Spice it up a bit with horseradish, which pairs nicely with caraway. In spring, substitute fresh peas or lightly steamed asparagus; replace the green beans with thinly sliced fennel in winter.

Peel the potatoes if you want. (We use organic potatoes so we usually leave the skin on.) Cut the potatoes into quarters, put them in a medium pot, and cover them with water. Add the salt to the water and cook the potatoes until they're tender but not too soft, about 15 minutes. Drain them and let them cool.

Meanwhile, bring a small pot of water to a boil. Boil the green beans until tender but still a bit crisp, about 3 minutes. Plunge them in cold water to stop the cooking, then drain them and let them cool.

Take the kraut out of the jar with a clean fork, letting any extra brine drain back into it. Roughly chop the kraut.

In a large bowl combine the cooled potatoes and green beans. Add the kraut, onions, radishes, parsley, and capers.

To make the dressing, in a small mixing bowl whisk together all the ingredients until well blended. Pour the dressing over the potato mixture and toss to coat. Serve immediately or refrigerate for up to 12 hours.

Makes 8 servings

8 medium red potatoes (about 2 pounds)

1 teaspoon salt

1 pound green beans, ends trimmed

1 cup Caraway Kraut (page 41)

¾ cup minced onion,

4 radishes, trimmed and minced

⅓ cup chopped fresh parsley

1 tablespoon capers, chopped (optional)

FOR THE DRESSING:

½ cup extra-virgin olive oil

2 tablespoons Dijon mustard

3 tablespoons apple cider vinegar

1 tablespoon mayonnaise or Greek yogurt

½ teaspoon caraway seeds, crushed

1 teaspoon salt

1 teaspoon horseradish (optional)

Kimchi Coleslaw

Coleslaw comes from the Dutch term koolsla, *which means "cool salad." Making cabbage cool is what we're all about, so why not add fermented cabbage to fresh cabbage and up the "cool" level and digestibility? The heat of Firefly Kimchi is just what classic coleslaw needs to brighten it up, plus the different textures of fresh and fermented cabbage keep it interesting.*

For a tasty egg-free alternative, omit the mayonnaise and add a splash of apple cider or rice wine vinegar and a tablespoon of sesame oil. Add shrimp, chicken, or tofu to boost the protein and turn the slaw into lunch or a light dinner.

Makes 4 to 6 servings

1 cup Firefly Kimchi (page 53)

4 green onions, chopped, including the green tops

½ small green or red cabbage, or a mix, shredded (about 4 cups)

2 to 3 medium carrots, grated (about 1 cup)

4 to 6 radished, trimmed and grated (about ½ cup)

Salt

FOR THE DRESSING:

½ cup mayonnaise or Greek yogurt

1 to 2 teaspoons of your favorite hot sauce

1 tablespoon freshly squeezed lime juice

1 tablespoon rice wine vinegar

Take the kimchi out of the jar with a clean fork, letting any extra brine drain back into it. Roughly chop the kimchi. Toss the kimchi with the remaining ingredients except the salt in a large bowl.

To make the dressing, whisk all the ingredients in a small bowl until well blended.

Pour the dressing over the slaw and toss to coat. Season to taste with salt. Serve immediately or refrigerate for up to 1 day.

Make It Quick & Simple

Brighten up your favorite coleslaw (or store-bought slaw) by topping it with the zesty flavor of your favorite kraut. The fermented cabbage will make the raw cabbage more digestible.

Queen Bean Salad

This colorful salad makes a great accompaniment to anything grilled and packs well for a picnic or barbecue. The combination of beans and avocados gives it a hearty, creamy consistency, peppered with the sweet crunch of bell peppers and corn, and the juiciness of tomatoes. The dish doubles as a great filler for tacos, burritos, and quesadillas.

Take the kraut out of the jar with a clean fork, letting any extra brine drain back into it. Roughly chop the kraut. Combine the kraut with the beans, bell pepper, corn, tomatoes, onion, cilantro, and jalapeño in a large mixing bowl.

To make the dressing, whisk all the ingredients in a small bowl until well mixed. Pour the dressing over the salad and toss to evenly coat. Season to taste with salt and pepper.

Top the salad with the avocado just before serving to keep it from getting brown. Serve chilled or at room temperature.

NOTE: Turn up the heat with a splash of your favorite salsa or an additional jalapeño.

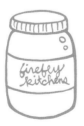

Makes 6 servings

1 cup Cortido Kraut (page 47)

1 (15-ounce) can white beans, rinsed and drained

1 (15-ounce) can black beans, rinsed and drained

1 (15-ounce) can kidney beans, rinsed and drained

2 large red bell peppers, cored, seeded, and diced (about 1½ cups)

1½ cups fresh corn kernels cut from the cob or frozen corn, thawed

1 cup halved cherry tomatoes

½ cup finely diced red onion

¼ cup chopped fresh cilantro

1 medium jalapeño, seeded and minced (about 3 tablespoons)

Salt and freshly ground black pepper

1 large avocado, halved, pitted, peeled, and diced

FOR THE DRESSING:

3 tablespoons red wine vinegar

1 teaspoon Dijon mustard

1 teaspoon cumin seeds, or ½ teaspoon ground cumin

½ teaspoon dried oregano

3 tablespoons extra-virgin olive oil

Pear, Fennel, and Pecan Salad

Make this salad when the trees take on rich hues of red and gold, and pears are at the peak of their season. Let them ripen until their flesh is tender to the touch. When you slice the pear just before serving, let its sweet juices run down into the greens and sweeten the entire salad. If you don't have a ripe pear on hand, try this with a sweet and crisp apple or four or five plump, juicy figs.

Makes 6 to 8 servings

¾ cup pecans

½ cup Ruby Red Kraut (page 43)

8 cups loosely packed baby greens (about 12 ounces)

½ medium fennel bulb, thinly sliced (about 1 cup)

½ cup crumbled blue cheese, such as Gorgonzola

FOR THE DRESSING:

¼ cup extra-virgin olive oil

2 tablespoons balsamic vinegar

1 teaspoon maple syrup

Salt and freshly ground black pepper

1 medium pear

In a small skillet over low heat, toast the pecans. Stir constantly (they burn easily) until they're browned and fragrant, 5 to 8 minutes.

Take the kraut out of the jar with a clean fork, letting any extra brine drain back into it. Roughly chop the kraut. In a large salad bowl, toss the kraut with the pecans, greens, fennel, and blue cheese.

To make the dressing, whisk all the ingredients in a small bowl until well blended.

Just before serving, drizzle the dressing over the greens and toss until it's evenly distributed. Season to taste with salt and pepper. Core and slice the pear, arrange the slices artfully on top of the salad, and serve immediately.

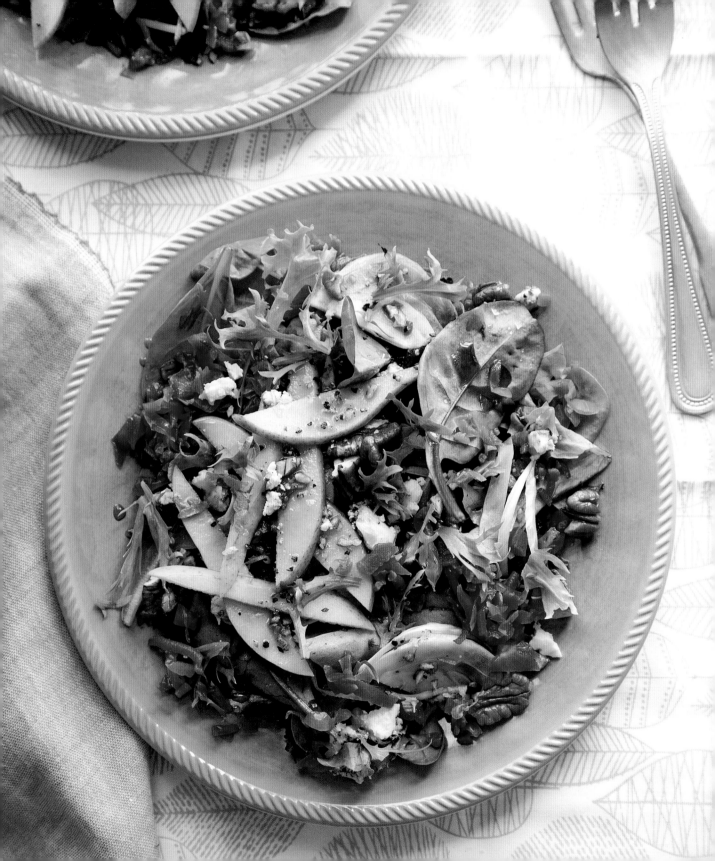

Firefly Chopped Salad

This hearty salad is a meal in itself or goes nicely with a light soup. We use different fruit and herb combinations depending on the season. In fall, we love to throw in thinly sliced apples, chopped fennel, or dried cherries to replace the dried apricots. For a creamier dressing, try adding a tablespoon or more of plain yogurt.

Makes 6 servings

1 cup Classic Kraut
(page 29)

1 cup chopped turkey cut into
½-inch cubes

½ cup chopped salami cut into
¼-inch cubes

1 cup (½ pound) mozzarella
cheese cut into ½-inch
cubes

1 red bell pepper, cored, seeded,
and diced (about ½ cup)

6 dried apricots, thinly sliced

⅓ cup chopped fresh parsley

1 head romaine lettuce, cored
and chopped into bite-size
pieces

FOR THE DRESSING:

1 teaspoon Dijon mustard

1 teaspoon maple syrup

¼ teaspoon smoked paprika
(*pimentón*)

Juice of 1 small lemon (about
2 tablespoons)

½ teaspoon salt

¼ cup extra-virgin olive oil

Remove the kraut from the jar with a fork, letting any extra brine drain back into the jar. Roughly chop the kraut. In a large salad bowl, toss the kraut with the turkey, salami, mozzarella, bell pepper, apricots, parsley, and lettuce. Refrigerate until ready to serve.

To make the dressing, whisk together all the ingredients except the oil in a small mixing bowl. Slowly drizzle in the oil, whisking constantly until the dressing is fully emulsified.

Just before serving, pour the dressing over the salad and toss to coat. Serve immediately.

Firefly Goddess Dressing

Creamy dressings make such a great addition to hearty salads, grains, and even roasted vegetables, but store-bought dressings are usually full of thickening agents and unhealthy fats. Our recipe relies on just a small amount of mayonnaise or plain yogurt to do the thickening and results in a fresh, light, and zesty dressing. Fresh herbs are key to its brightness—feel free to play around with seasonal herbs.

Use this to dress your favorite greens, coleslaw, or grain salad, or use it as a dip for vegetables or chips. We also love to pour it over baked potatoes and steamed broccoli.

Whirl all the ingredients except the salt and pepper in a blender or food processor until smooth. Season to taste with salt and pepper. Refrigerate until ready to use, and store this dressing in the fridge for up to 3 to 5 days.

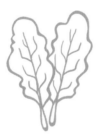

Makes about 3 cups

1 clove garlic, crushed

¾ cup Classic Kraut (page 29)

1 tablespoon apple cider vinegar

½ cup mayonnaise or plain Greek or whole-milk yogurt

¾ cup chopped fresh basil

¾ cup chopped fresh parsley

½ cup chopped fresh cilantro

¼ cup chopped, stemmed kale leaves

¼ teaspoon salt

¼ teaspoon sugar

¼ teaspoon lime zest

1 teaspoon freshly squeezed lime juice

Salt and freshly ground black pepper

Everyday Everyway Dressing

As its name suggests, this is a simple, go-to dressing that will quickly become a standard in your kitchen. Simple to make, it's versatile enough to work well with a wide variety of ingredients, including all Firefly ferments. Make a big batch and keep it on hand to dress a bowl of greens or drizzle over veggies or grains for a quick and healthy meal.

Makes about 2 cups

3 cloves garlic, crushed and finely chopped

2 tablespoons water

1 tablespoon Dijon or stone-ground mustard

1 tablespoons tamari

⅓ cup apple cider vinegar

1 tablespoon honey or maple syrup

1 cup extra-virgin olive oil

1 teaspoon salt

½ teaspoon freshly ground black pepper

Put the garlic, water, mustard, tamari, vinegar, and honey in a pint jar with a lid that screws on tight. Secure the lid and shake the jar vigorously for 30 seconds, or until the ingredients are well mixed.

Add the oil, secure the lid again, and shake the jar for another 30 seconds, or until the ingredients are well mixed. Season to taste with salt and pepper. Store this dressing on your kitchen counter or in the fridge for up to two weeks.

STRAIGHT UP

If you have any brine left after you've eaten all the kraut, it works well in place of vinegar in most recipes, especially salad dressings, and some people love to drink it straight from the jar.

Chapter 8:
Sandwiches, Wraps & Burgers

Hearty Lettuce Cups

We designed these cups as another quick meal you can put together with the leftovers you have on hand. Delicate butter leaf lettuce makes a fun vehicle for this incredibly flavorful filling of meat, chicken, fish, or tofu and veggies.

You can also get creative with the filling—mix and match proteins and seasonal veggies, or try incorporating grains or legumes instead. Top each lettuce cup with extra kimchi, any of your favorite krauts, or Yin Yang Carrots (page 55) for an extra splash of flavor and crunch.

Makes 18 to 24 lettuce cups

1 tablespoon coconut oil or butter

1 small yellow onion, diced (about 1 cup)

½ teaspoon salt

6 medium mushrooms, diced

3 cups cooked leftover meat, tofu, or other protein

1 to 2 medium carrots, grated (about ¾ cup)

¼ cup chopped fresh cilantro

2 tablespoons chopped fresh mint (optional)

FOR THE SAUCE:

2 tablespoons coconut oil or butter

1 cup Firefly Kimchi (page 53)

2 tablespoons apple cider vinegar

½ cup cashews, chopped

Juice of 1 medium lime (about 2 tablespoons)

2 teaspoons honey

2 tablespoons tamari

2 to 4 tablespoons water, to thin (if needed)

16 to 20 medium leaves butter leaf or red leaf lettuce (from 1 to 2 heads lettuce)

Heat the coconut oil in a large sauté pan over medium heat. Add the onions and salt, and sauté until the onions are translucent, about 10 minutes. Add the mushrooms and sauté until their moisture has evaporated, about 5 minutes.

Transfer the mushrooms and onions to a large mixing bowl. Add the meat, carrots, cilantro, and mint, and thoroughly combine.

To make the sauce, combine all the ingredients except the water in a blender or food processor, and whirl until smooth. If it's too thick, add water, 1 tablespoon at a time, until the sauce is the consistency you want. Pour the sauce over the veggie mixture and toss to combine.

Scoop a small amount of the protein and veggie mixture into the center of each lettuce leaf and arrange the leaves on a serving platter, or serve the mixture with lettuce leaves on the side so your guests can make their own wraps.

Cortuna Collard Wraps

Cortido Kraut + tuna = Cortuna.

This wrap starts with a tuna salad punctuated with tangy kraut. Steamed collards add a healthy lining to your favorite tortilla. These wraps are great as a light lunch or portable snack, but you could also turn them into an appetizer by slicing the wrap and skewering the slices with toothpicks to keep them rolled up.

Bring a large pot of water to a rapid boil. With a sharp knife, remove the thick stems of the collards, keeping the leaves whole. Drop the collards into the boiling water and cook until they are just wilted, about 1 minute. Remove the collards, quickly rinse them with cold water to stop the cooking, drain them, and set them aside.

Drain the liquid from the cans of tuna and put the tuna in a medium mixing bowl. Take the kraut out of the jar with a clean fork, letting any extra brine drain back into it. Roughly chop the kraut and add it to the tuna, along with the mayonnaise, celery, bell pepper, and red pepper flakes, and mix well. Season to taste with salt and pepper.

To make the wrap, put a tortilla on a work surface and lay a collard leaf on top of the tortilla. Scoop ¼ of the tuna mixture onto each collard and tightly roll it up burrito-style.

Serve immediately or refrigerate for up to 3 hours before serving.

Makes 4 wraps

4 medium collard leaves

2 (5-ounce) cans wild-caught tuna

1 cup Cortido Kraut (page 47)

¼ cup mayonnaise

⅓ cup finely diced celery

½ cup finely diced red bell pepper (½ small pepper)

½ teaspoon red pepper flakes (optional)

Salt and freshly ground black pepper

4 (8-inch) flour or corn tortillas

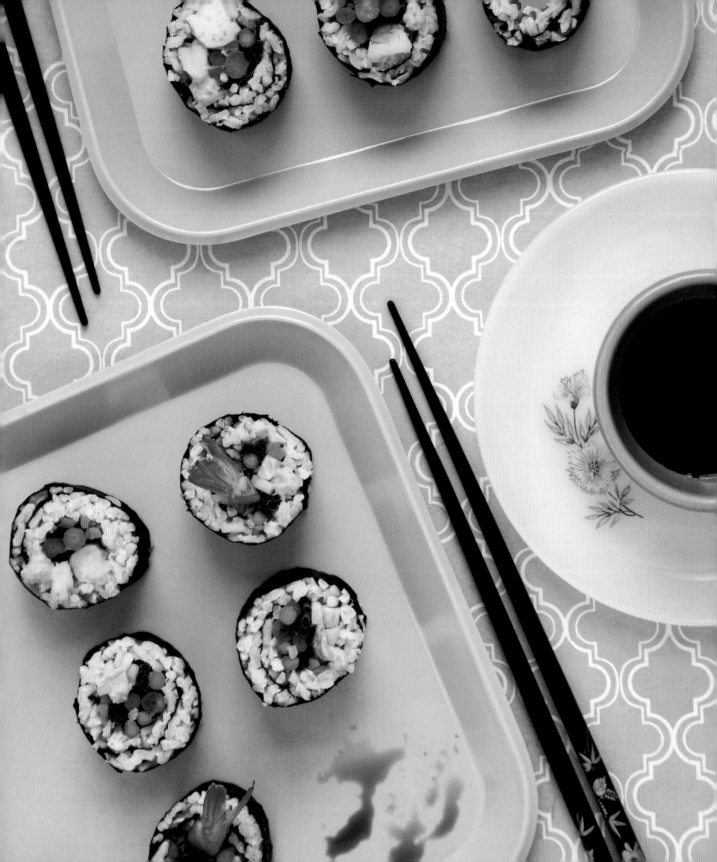

Sauerkraut Sushi

Satisfying, fun, and surprisingly simple, making sushi at home allows you to completely customize every roll to your taste and texture preferences. Make it as spicy, crunchy, colorful, simple, or complex as you like by choosing your own fillings. We've included some of our favorites below, but avocado, radishes, sautéed mushrooms, cilantro, cooked or raw sushi-grade fish (make sure it's fresh!), and tofu also make great additions.

To make the sauce, take the kraut out of the jar with a clean fork, letting any extra brine drain back into it. Put the kraut, avocado, mayonnaise, wasabi, and soy sauce in a blender or food processor and whirl until smooth. Set aside.

Cut the cucumber lengthwise into 8 pieces. (Slicing this and the other veggies lengthwise makes it easier to build a tidy sushi roll.) Using a vegetable peeler, shave the length of the carrot to make ribbons.

To prepare the wraps, fill a small bowl with hot water and place it next to your work surface. Lay a sheet of nori on a flexible surface, such as a bamboo sushi rolling mat or a tea towel lined with plastic wrap. Spread about ½ cup of the rice evenly over the nori, leaving about an inch of exposed nori on the far edge. Spread 1 to 2 teaspoons of the prepared sauce on the rice. Lay 1 cucumber piece, a few carrot ribbons, ½ green onion, 1 asparagus spear, and 3 prawn halves lengthwise across the rice. Moisten the exposed nori on the far edge with a little warm water from your bowl.

continued

Makes 8 rolls

- 1½ cups Classic Kraut (page 29)
- 1 large avocado, halved, pitted, and peeled
- 1 tablespoon mayonnaise or cream cheese
- ½ to 1 teaspoon powdered wasabi
- ½ to 1 teaspoon soy sauce or tamari, plus extra soy sauce for serving
- 1 medium cucumber, peeled
- 2 medium carrots
- 8 (8-by-8-inch) sheets nori
- 4 cups cooked brown rice (see Rice, page 214, for cooking instructions)
- 4 green onions, sliced in half lengthwise
- 8 to 10 asparagus spears, steamed (optional)
- 12 medium prawns, cooked and sliced in half down the midline (optional)
- Pickled ginger, for serving (optional)

Starting with the rice- and veggie-covered edge, roll the nori around the filling until the rice is enclosed and the moistened seaweed edge seals the roll. Gently squeeze the roll evenly. Unroll the nori from the bamboo roller or plastic wrap and set aside. Repeat the filling and rolling process with the remaining nori sheets.

When you're ready to slice your rolls, dip a sharp knife in hot water (to prevent it from sticking), and slice each roll crosswise into about 8 pieces.

Serve with soy sauce and any remaining wasabi kraut sauce for dipping. Pickled ginger also makes a great accompaniment.

NORI IS GOOD FOR YOU

As a nutrient-dense food, nori (seaweed) is a rare source of vitamin B_{12}, which is necessary for energy production; other B vitamins; vitamins C and E; iodine; and numerous trace minerals that benefit the body.

Fresh Spring Rolls

Fresh and crunchy, these gluten-free, vegan, and paleo-friendly burrito-style rolls are perfect for a packed lunch or as a light dinner or refreshing appetizer. Almost any vegetable you have on hand will work well, so get creative with combinations. For a dipping sauce variation, try mixing a tablespoon of hoisin sauce into a ½ cup of our PB Chi Spread (page 105). Spring rolls make a great meal on their own when you add cooked and thinly sliced prawns, chicken, beef, or tofu to the filling.

Put the vermicelli in a medium heatproof bowl. Pour the boiling water over the noodles until they're submerged, and let them sit until they're soft but not mushy, 2 to 3 minutes. Stir once to keep them from clumping. Drain the noodles, rinse them with cold water to stop the cooking, and set them aside to cool.

Fill a pie pan with warm water. Soak a sheet of the rice paper in the water until it softens, about 30 seconds. With your hands (not a utensil, lest it tear the paper), carefully transfer the sheet from the water to a cutting board or large plate.

Make each roll right after you remove the rice paper from the water. Put about 1 tablespoon of the vermicelli on a rice paper round. Add about 2 tablespoons each of the carrots, jicama, and greens, and an herb sprig. Tightly roll up the rice paper burrito-style. (The rice paper will naturally stick to itself, sealing the roll.)

Put the roll seam side down on a serving plate and prepare the remaining rolls. Once all the wraps are prepared, slice them in half on the diagonal.

To make the dipping sauce, combine all the ingredients in a small bowl, stirring well. Pour the sauce into a serving bowl and serve with the wraps.

Makes 8 rolls

2 ounces rice vermicelli

4 cups boiling water

8 large round sheets of rice paper, also called spring roll wrappers

1 cup Yin Yang Carrots (page 55)

1 cup (½ medium) grated jicama

2 cups chopped spinach or greens of your choice

8 sprigs fresh herbs, such as mint, basil, or cilantro

FOR THE DIPPING SAUCE:

¼ cup rice wine vinegar

¼ cup tamari

1 tablespoon honey

2 teaspoons sesame oil

2 cloves garlic, crushed

1 teaspoon minced fresh ginger

1 teaspoon toasted sesame seeds (optional)

Egg Salad Sandwiches 3 Ways

Kraut and eggs are the ultimate power couple. Kraut provides the probiotics and enzymes to help you digest the protein-rich eggs, and the hint of tangy brine enlivens the eggs' creaminess. When you're serving a crowd, make more than one egg salad so your guests have a few flavor combinations to choose from.

Keep the sandwich simple by spreading mayonnaise on the bread, or, for a little variety, Dijon mustard, aioli, or Sun-Dried Tomato Tapenade (page 104) are great choices. We always like adding a slice or two of tomato when they're in season and finish with lettuce. You can make this as an open-faced sandwich too.

You could easily turn these egg salads into deviled eggs for a more elegant occasion or serve the egg salad in a creative way, wrapping it in lettuce leaves or spooning into hollowed-out cucumber halves.

Makes 2 to 4 servings

4 hard-boiled organic eggs, peeled

2 tablespoons mayonnaise

½ teaspoon salt

¼ teaspoon freshly ground black pepper

½ cup Firefly Kimchi (page 53)

4 to 8 slices whole-wheat or hearty French bread

Condiments of your choice (such as mayonnaise, mustard, aioli, or tapenade)

Tomato slices and lettuce leaves, for serving (optional)

The Basic

Put the eggs, mayonnaise, salt, and pepper in a medium bowl. Smash the eggs with the back of a fork, breaking them down into small chunks. Take the kimchi out of the jar with a clean fork, letting any extra brine drain back into it. Dice the kimchi and add it to the egg mixture and stir to combine the ingredients.

Spread 2 to 4 slices of bread with your preferred condiment, spread ¼ to ½ of the egg salad (depending on how many sandwiches you're making) on the bread, add the tomato and lettuce, top with the remaining 2 to 4 bread slices, and serve immediately. The egg salad can be made ahead and refrigerated for up to 24 hours.

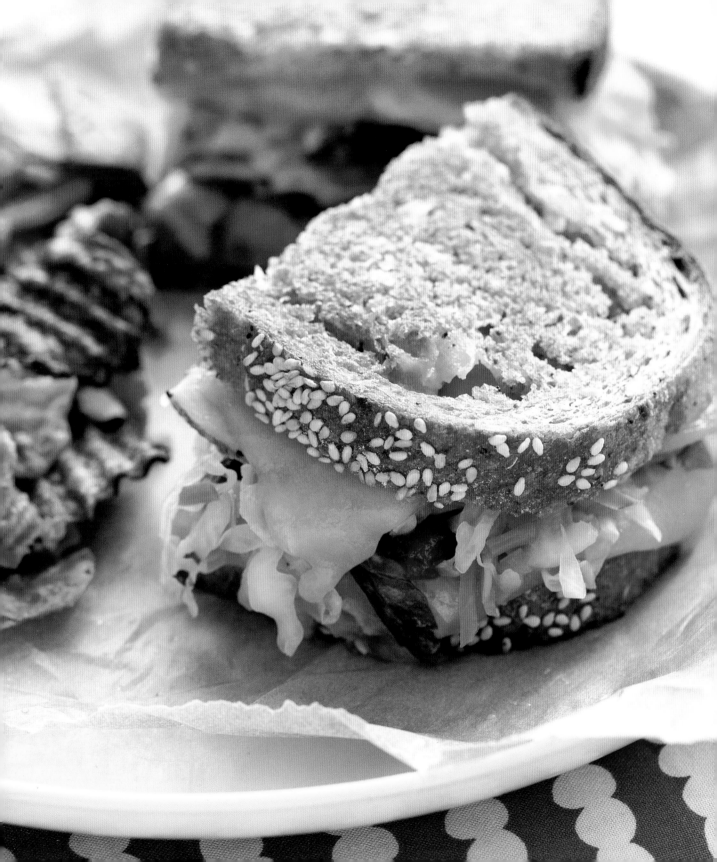

Smoked Salmon Reuben

In Seattle, we are fortunate to have many chefs who are dedicated to local, seasonal, and sustainable whole foods. Cynthia Lair—chef, nutrition educator, and hilarious improv actor—is one of our favorite local food celebrities. Cynthia's first book, Feeding the Whole Family, *has been a solid resource for our cooking and has provided much inspiration for the creations at Firefly Kitchens. She was kind enough to share her grilled Smoked Salmon Reuben recipe. It's also fantastic made with Caraway Kraut (page 41) instead of Classic Kraut and pastrami in place of the salmon.*

Makes 4 sandwiches

1 cup Classic Kraut (page 29)

8 slices rye or whole-grain sourdough bread

4 slices Havarti or Swiss cheese

½ pound smoked salmon, thinly sliced

2 tablespoons pickle relish (optional)

2 tablespoons ketchup (optional)

2 tablespoons mayonnaise (optional)

2 tablespoons whole-grain mustard (optional)

4 teaspoons butter, divided

Take the kraut out of the jar with a clean fork, letting any extra brine drain back into it. Roughly chop the kraut. On one piece of bread, add a slice of cheese followed by ¼ of the salmon, then add the condiments to the second piece of bread. Repeat for the additional sandwiches.

Heat 2 teaspoons of the butter in a large skillet over medium heat. Put two sandwiches in the skillet, and cook until one side of the bread is golden and toasted, 3 to 4 minutes. Flip the sandwiches, and repeat on the other side. Remove the sandwiches from the pan and set them aside. Put the remaining butter in the skillet and cook the remaining two sandwiches in the same manner.

Cut each sandwich in half and serve right away.

Krauty Joes

When Denise Breyley, Whole Foods Market's West Coast Forager, called us for a Super Bowl recipe to put on her blog, the occasion seemed right for sloppy joes. Our version has less sugar than traditional recipes and a heaping dose of tangy kraut to balance the rich sauce and fuel the digestive fire. Try maple syrup or molasses (or a combo) instead of brown sugar and see what you think.

Heat the oil in a large skillet over medium heat. Add the onion and sauté until translucent, about 10 minutes. Add the bell pepper and garlic and sauté for another 2 minutes. Add the beef and sauté, stirring frequently, until it's cooked through, 7 to 9 minutes. Stir in the tomato sauce, tomato paste, vinegar, brown sugar, and mustard, and cook until all the ingredients are hot and bubbly, 5 to 7 minutes. Thin the mixture with the water, 2 tablespoons at a time, to get the consistency you like. Season to taste with salt and pepper.

Toast the buns if you want to. Spoon ¼ of the sloppy joe mixture onto the base of each bun. Top each with ¼ cup kraut. Place the other half of the bun on top and serve hot.

Makes 4 servings

- 1 teaspoon olive or coconut oil
- ½ cup finely diced onion
- ⅓ cup finely diced green bell pepper
- 2 cloves garlic, minced
- 1 pound grass-fed ground beef
- 1½ cups tomato sauce
- 1 tablespoon tomato paste
- 2 teaspoons apple cider vinegar
- 2 tablespoons packed brown sugar
- 1 tablespoon Dijon mustard
- 2 tablespoons water or more as needed
- Salt and freshly ground black pepper
- 4 burger buns, or 8 slices hearty sourdough bread
- 1 cup Classic Kraut (page 29)

Triple-B Veggie Burgers

In many Asian countries, the nutty and sweet adzuki bean is used in desserts. Here, we combine them with beets, leftover rice, and Ruby Red Kraut to create a very "meaty" vegetarian patty. It's the beans, beets, and brown rice that give this dish its name. Meat eater–approved, these burgers will be the star of a summer barbecue.

Make a double batch and freeze any extra patties for a quick lunch or dinner down the road. The burgers cook well both in a heavy cast-iron pan and on the grill.

Makes 4 servings

2 tablespoons extra-virgin olive oil or butter, divided

½ small white onion, finely diced (about ½ cup)

1 teaspoon ground cumin

1 teaspoon chili powder

½ small red beet, shredded (about ½ cup)

1½ cups cooked adzuki or black beans (see Legumes, page 215, for cooking instructions), or 1 (15-ounce) can, drained

1 cup cooked brown rice (see Rice, page 214, for cooking instructions)

2 teaspoons salt

1 teaspoon freshly ground black pepper

½ cup Ruby Red Kraut (page 43)

2 organic eggs, beaten

⅔ cup all-purpose flour

4 burger buns

Heat 1 tablespoon of the oil in a medium skillet over medium-low heat. Add the onion and sauté until translucent, about 10 minutes. Add the cumin and chili powder, stir, and cook until the spices are fragrant, another minute. Put the spiced onions into a large mixing bowl. Do not clean the skillet—you will use it later.

Mix the beets, beans, rice, salt, and pepper into the onions. Take the kraut out of the jar with a clean fork, letting any extra brine drain back into it. Roughly chop the kraut and add it to the beet mixture. Add the eggs and mix to incorporate. Add the flour, a few spoonfuls at a time, stirring after each addition. The mixture should soon clump together into a sticky, but moldable, consistency. Form the mixture into 4 large patties.

Heat the remaining 1 tablespoon oil over medium heat in the skillet you used for the onions. Place the burgers in the pan and cook until they're lightly crisp and toasted on one side, 4 to 5 minutes. Flip the burgers and repeat, this time covering the pan. Cook until browned, about 10 or so minutes.

Place each burger on a bun, garnish with your toppings of choice—of course, kraut is great on burgers. Serve immediately.

SuperKraut Burgers

Burgers are a classic and ideal vehicle to load up with all sorts of kraut and other toppings. We couldn't pick which ones to share, so we give you one basic burger and three different topping variations depending on the kraut you choose.

The Basic

However you plan on cooking your burgers, heat things up: pre-heat the barbecue, stove-top griddle, or oven (to 375 degrees F).

Combine all the burger ingredients in a large bowl and knead them together until well incorporated. Form the meat mixture into 4 patties.

Cook the patties for 4 to 5 minutes on one side. Flip the burgers and cook until they're done the way you like them.

While the burgers are cooking, toast the buns. Put each patty on a freshly toasted bun, add the toppings of your choice, and serve hot.

continued

Makes 4 burgers

1 pound grass-fed ground beef

1 teaspoon Dijon mustard

½ teaspoon garlic powder

½ teaspoon freshly ground black pepper

½ teaspoon salt

1 teaspoon Worcestershire sauce (optional)

4 burger buns

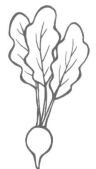

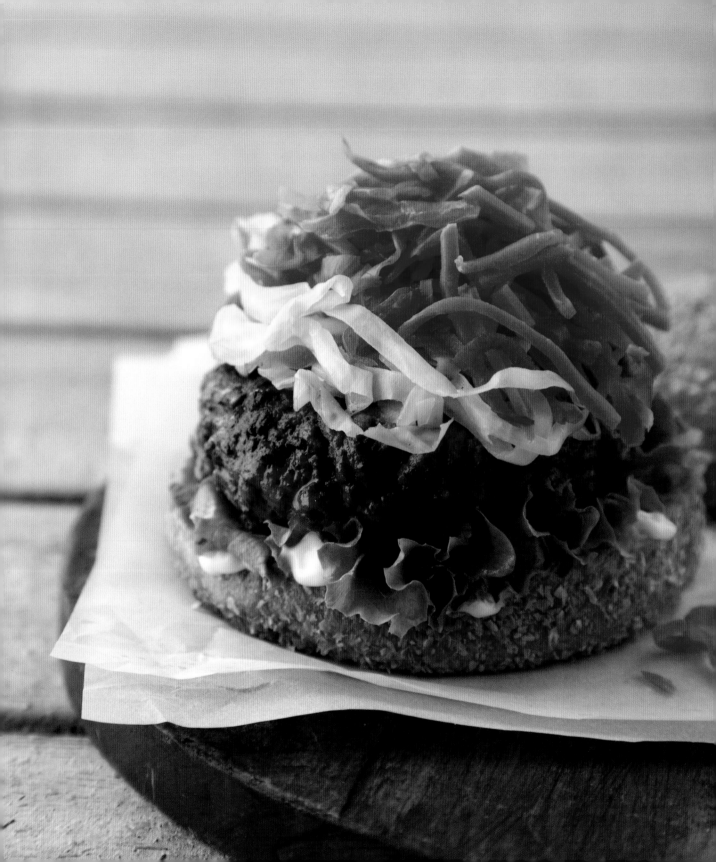

Variations

SUPER KIMCHI BURGER: Top each burger with about ⅓ cup Firefly Kimchi (page 53), sliced avocado, a fried egg, and a small handful of fresh spinach.

SUPER CARAWAY BURGER: Top each burger with mayonnaise, Dijon mustard, about ⅓ cup Caraway Kraut (page 41), a small handful of sprouts, and a slice of cheddar cheese.

SUPER RUBY RED BURGER: Top each burger with about ⅓ cup Ruby Red Kraut (page 43), sliced avocado, a couple slices of cooked bacon, and a few thin slices of tomato.

KRAUTIFY YOUR CONDIMENTS

While we've heard some folks call our krauts "the little black dress of condiments," we like to think of them as necessary ingredients for a well-balanced meal. Here's a list of classic American condiments and a simple way to "krautify" them so you get your daily dose of beneficial bacteria—and good flavor!

The easiest way to make these a bit more zesty and interesting is to simply mix a teaspoon or two of minced Classic Kraut (page 29) into each serving of your favorite condiment. If you have a jar of Classic Kraut blended up, that will make adding kraut even faster. Try with these condiments:

- Salsa
- Ketchup
- Mustard
- Barbecue sauce
- Tartar sauce
- Mayonnaise
- Horseradish
- Pickle relish
- Hot sauce
- Sweet and sour sauce
- Steak sauce

Chapter 9:
Veggies & Grains: Sides or Solo

Tri-Way Cabbage Sauté

There's no such thing as too much cabbage in our world. Fresh, sautéed, and fermented cabbage all work well in combination, and each one complements the other with additional texture, flavor, and health benefits. With this medley of sautéed cabbage, vegetables, spices, and krauts we hope to provide you with a variety of side dish options that are quick, easy, and accessible.

Gluten-free, vegan, nutrient-rich, and versatile, these three cabbage sautés can be put together at the last minute and make excellent additions to grilled meats and fish. They're also a great way to quickly put together a main meal for those with dietary restrictions. They work well in place of pasta, served with your favorite sauce, or substituted for any grain with the dressing of your choice. Mix and match flavors, krauts, and vegetables—try different cabbages—and add shredded chicken, sliced prawns, or diced tofu to the mix.

Makes about 3 cups

2 tablespoons coconut or extra-virgin olive oil

4 cups shredded green cabbage (about ⅔ pound)

1 teaspoon ground turmeric

½ to 1 cup Emerald City Kraut (page 49)

Salt and freshly ground black pepper

The Basic

Heat the oil in a large sauté pan over medium heat. Add the cabbage and sauté until wilted, 5 to 8 minutes. Add the turmeric and sauté until fragrant, another 3 to 4 minutes.

Remove the pan from the heat and let the cabbage cool for a few minutes. Take the kraut out of the jar using a clean fork, letting any extra brine drain back into it, then roughly chop the kraut. Add the kraut to the cabbage, toss to combine, and season to taste with salt and pepper. Serve immediately.

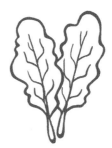

Variations

RAINBOW SAUTÉ

Heat the oil in a large sauté pan over medium heat. Add the cabbage and sauté until wilted, 5 to 8 minutes. Add the chard, beets, carrots, and green onions, and sauté until soft, another 3 to 4 minutes.

Remove the pan from the heat and let the vegetables cool for a few minutes. Toss with the kraut, and season to taste with salt and pepper. Serve immediately.

GREEN SAUTÉ

Heat the oil in a large sauté pan over medium heat. Add the onions and sauté until translucent, about 10 minutes. Add the garlic and sauté until golden for another 2 minutes. Add the cabbage and sauté until wilted, 5 to 6 minutes. Add the kale and sauté until wilted for another 3 to 4 minutes, stirring to incorporate.

Remove the pan from the heat and let the greens cool for a few minutes. Toss with the kraut, and season to taste with salt and pepper. Serve immediately.

FOR THE RAINBOW SAUTÉ:

2 tablespoons coconut or extra-virgin olive oil

4 cups shredded green cabbage, sliced chiffonade (about ⅔ pound)

1 cup shredded rainbow chard

½ small red beet, shredded (about ½ cups)

3 to 4 medium carrots, grated (about 1½ cups)

4 green onions, sliced, including the green tops

½ to 1 cup Ruby Red Kraut (page 43)

Salt and freshly ground black pepper

FOR THE GREEN SAUTÉ:

2 tablespoons coconut or extra-virgin olive oil

1 small white or yellow onion, sliced

3 cloves garlic, minced

4 cups shredded green cabbage (about ⅔ pound)

2 cups stemmed and thinly sliced kale or beet greens

½ to 1 cup Caraway Kraut (page 41)

Salt and freshly ground black pepper

Scarlet Millet

Mildly nutty, and naturally gluten-free, millet is an ancient seed that is cooked and eaten as you would a grain. When cooked it becomes a soft and fluffy delicacy that pairs well with just about anything. In this recipe, the millet takes on a vibrant magenta color and a sweet earthy flavor from the raw beets, making this a spectacular side dish to serve with less vividly colored foods such as halibut, chicken, or tofu. Jazz it up by stirring in feta cheese, toasted nuts, pumpkin seeds, green onions, or chives at the end.

Makes 4 to 8 servings

1 cup millet

2 cups water

1 cup Ruby Red Kraut
(page 43)

1 medium red beet, shredded
(about 1 cup)

Zest of 1 lemon

Juice of 1 medium lemon
(about 3 tablespoons)

3 tablespoons extra-virgin
olive oil or flaxseed oil

3 tablespoons finely chopped
fresh mint, basil, or parsley

Salt and freshly ground black
pepper

Toast the millet in a large dry saucepan over medium heat until you hear it start to pop, 4 to 5 minutes. Immediately add the water to the pan and bring it to a boil. Reduce the heat slightly, cover the pan, and simmer the millet for 15 minutes.

Remove the pan from the heat and let it rest with the cover on for 10 minutes. Transfer the millet to a large serving bowl and use a fork to fluff it and break up any clumps.

Take the kraut out of the jar using a clean fork, letting any extra brine drain back into it. Roughly chop the kraut, and add it to the millet. Mix in the beets, lemon zest, lemon juice, oil, and mint. Season to taste with salt and pepper and serve immediately, or refrigerate for up to 2 hours before serving.

> **NOTE:** If you want to keep Scarlet Millet on hand for a few days for lunches or snacks, wait to add the kraut and oil. Everything else can be mixed together before refrigeration. Spoon a dollop of kraut on top and drizzle with oil just before you're ready to eat.

Caraway-Kale-Cauliflower Fluff

Perfect for a crisp fall day or chilly winter evening, this dish offers the comforting sensations of a rich casserole as well as the health benefits of nutrient-packed cruciferous vegetables. We particularly love dinosaur (aka lacinato) kale in this recipe.

This dish is a great way to sneak extra veggies into your diet and makes an excellent accompaniment to roast chicken or turkey, grilled sausage, or a hearty roast.

Preheat the oven to 350 degrees F.

Steam the cauliflower until it's soft and tender, 5 to 8 minutes. Set it aside.

Melt the butter over low heat in a small sauté pan. Add the garlic and cook until it's golden and fragrant, about 1 minute. Add the kale and salt, and sauté until the kale is just wilted, another 2 to 3 minutes.

Transfer the kale mixture to a food processor and pulse until it's finely chopped. Add the cauliflower and whirl until the mixture is smooth. Add the kraut and pepper, and pulse until the kraut is well mixed in, but small pieces still remain. (If you don't have a food processor, mash it by hand as you would potatoes—it will be a little chunkier.)

Sprinkle the Parmesan evenly over the top. Check for seasoning and add more salt and pepper if needed. Serve hot with additional kraut as a garnish.

Makes 4 to 6 servings

- 1 medium cauliflower (about 2 pounds), cut into 1-inch florets
- ¼ cup (½ stick) unsalted butter
- 3 to 5 medium cloves garlic, minced
- 1 cup stemmed and thinly sliced kale
- 1 teaspoon salt
- ½ cup Caraway Kraut (page 41), plus extra for garnish
- ½ teaspoon freshly ground black pepper
- ½ cup grated Parmesan cheese (about 2 ounces) (optional)

Yin Yang Yams

This is a super side dish, slightly sweet but hearty and comforting, with a whopping dose of vitamin C, potassium, and fiber. It's fancy enough to serve on Thanksgiving or holidays, yet casual enough for a weeknight meal, and so easy to prepare that it will quickly become a staple. Kids love the earthy sweetness of yams so this recipe is a great way to sneak a lot of nutrients, as well as some fermented vegetables, into their diet. (Adults might want to double the amount of Yin Yang Carrots for a more savory flavor.)

Speaking of sweetness, with a little doctoring, this dish can double as a healthy dessert. Add some cinnamon, maple syrup, and heavy cream or coconut milk to the whirl, and serve it with a dollop of ice cream or a sprinkling of cinnamon sugar.

Makes about 2 cups

1 large or 2 small yams
(about 1 pound)

2 to 3 tablespoons coconut oil, melted

2 tablespoons unsweetened dried coconut flakes

⅓ cup Yin Yang Carrots (page 55)

Salt

Preheat the oven to 350 degrees F.

Scrub the yam to remove any dirt and prick the skin a few times with the tip of a knife. (This allows moisture to escape during cooking without causing the skin to burst.) Bake the yam on a baking sheet or in a baking dish until it's soft all the way through (test this by piercing it with a knife), about 35 minutes. Remove the yam and set it aside until it's cool enough to handle.

When the yam has cooled, cut it in half and use a large spoon to scoop out the flesh. Discard the skin, and put the flesh in a food processor. Add the coconut oil and coconut flakes and blend until the yam mixture is smooth, about 1 minute. Add the carrots and blend until they're finely chopped and well incorporated, about 1 minute. Season to taste with salt. Serve immediately, topping with additional Yin Yang Carrots if you want.

NOTE: If you don't have a food processor, mash the yams by hand as you would potatoes, and simply stir in the coconut oil, coconut flakes, and carrots.

Stuffed Zucchini Boats

This recipe takes a little extra time to prepare, but its rich flavor and texture are worth it. It can stand alone as a vegetarian main meal or serve as the perfect side to grilled fish or chicken. It can also double as an appetizer if you cut it into 1-inch pieces. Any grain you have on hand will be tasty in this dish, including quinoa, wild rice, and bulgur wheat.

Preheat the oven to 350 degrees F.

Scoop out the flesh of each zucchini half, leaving about ¼ inch on the sides and bottom to maintain stability. Finely chop the flesh.

Heat the oil in a medium sauté pan over medium heat. Add the chopped zucchini and sauté until it softens and its moisture evaporates, 4 to 5 minutes. Add the garlic and sauté until fragrant, 2 to 3 minutes. Take the kimchi out of the jar with a clean fork, letting any extra brine drain back into it. Roughly chop the kimchi and add it to the zucchini sauté. Mix in the rice and goat cheese, and stir until the cheese has melted, 3 to 4 minutes. Remove the pan from the heat.

Put the zucchini boats in a 9-by-13-inch baking dish. Spoon about ½ cup of the rice mixture into each zucchini, spreading it evenly. Add 1 to 2 tablespoons of water to the bottom of the baking dish. Bake until the zucchini are soft and the filling is hot, 15 to 20 minutes.

Garnish each boat with about 2 tablespoons of the kimchi and serve hot.

Makes 4 to 8 servings

3 tablespoons extra-virgin olive oil

4 medium zucchini (about 1½ pounds), sliced in half lengthwise

3 cloves garlic, chopped

½ cup Firefly Kimchi (page 53), plus about 1 cup for serving (optional)

1 cup cooked brown rice (see Rice, page 214, for cooking instructions)

⅔ cup crumbled goat cheese (about 3 ounces)

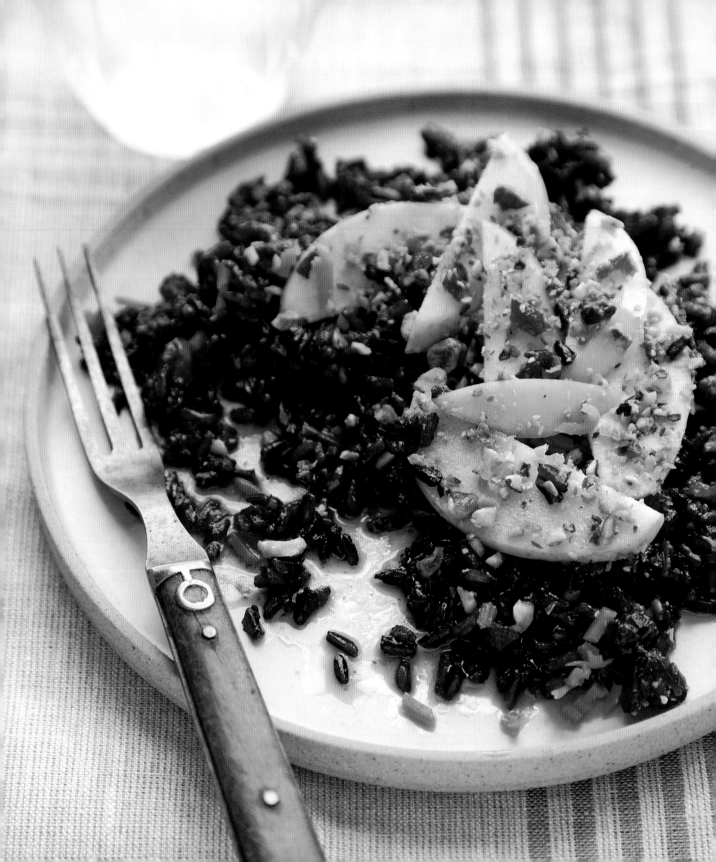

Not-So-Forbidden Rice

Legends tell that this beautiful black rice was once eaten only by Chinese emperors, who didn't allow the general public to consume it—thus the name "forbidden rice." Said to bring health and longevity to those who ate it, it was a highly prized commodity. At least part of its history stands true: research shows that black rice is one of the most nutrient-rich rice varieties—it's high in antioxidants, iron, and magnesium.

When cooked, the rice's almost-black color turns to a gorgeous deep purple that is stunning in contrast to the vibrant orange carrots in this dish. Its nutty, sweet flavors are accentuated by dried and fresh fruit and nuts. Notes of fall permeate the simple dressing.

This dish is a striking accompaniment to any white fish or roast chicken. Roasted squash, dried cherries, or other toasted nuts work well as additions or substitutions.

Take the carrots out of the jar with a clean fork, letting any extra brine drain back into it. Roughly chop the carrots and put them in a large bowl. Mix in the rice, cranberries, pistachios, and apples.

In a small bowl, whisk the cinnamon, salt, oil, vinegar, and maple syrup until smooth. Pour the mixture over the rice and toss to incorporate.

Serve immediately or refrigerate for a few hours to serve chilled.

Makes 6 to 8 servings

1 cup Yin Yang Carrots (page 55)

3 cups cooked black rice, cooled (see Rice, page 214, for cooking instructions)

½ cup dried cranberries, chopped

½ cup shelled pistachios, chopped

1 medium apple, cored, and cut into ¼-inch pieces

¼ teaspoon ground cinnamon

½ teaspoon salt

⅓ cup extra-virgin olive oil

2 tablespoons apple cider vinegar

2 teaspoons maple syrup

Roasted Eggplant and Farro

This recipe came from our fantastic intern, Nora Dummer, a Bastyr University graduate. It calls for pearled farro, which takes less time to cook than whole-grain or semi-pearled, but if you'd like to up the nutritional value, use whole-grain farro and be sure to soak it overnight.

The simplicity of this dish makes it versatile, forgiving, and easy to modify. Use grilled eggplant rather than baked, add fresh tomatoes or other seasonal vegetables, or use any kraut of your choice to make this dish your own. It makes an excellent accompaniment to Halibut with Avocado Butter (page 183) or roast chicken.

Makes about 4 cups

1 large eggplant

2 teaspoons salt

1 cup pearled farro

1¾ cups vegetable stock or water

¼ cup pine nuts

3 tablespoons extra-virgin olive oil, divided

½ cup Classic Kraut (page 29)

3 cloves garlic, minced

Zest of 1 lemon

Juice of 1 medium lemon (about 3 tablespoons)

1 cup finely chopped fresh basil

Salt and freshly ground black pepper

Cut off the stem end of the eggplant and cut it into ¾-inch cubes. Put the cubes in a colander and sprinkle them with the salt, tossing to coat. Let the cubes rest for at least 30 minutes to release their moisture.

Meanwhile, put the farro and stock in a small saucepan and bring the stock to a boil over high heat. Lower the heat, cover, and simmer until the liquid is absorbed and the farro is soft but still fairly chewy, 15 to 20 minutes. Transfer the farro to a large bowl to cool.

While the farro is cooking, toast the pine nuts in a small skillet over low heat. Stir constantly (they burn easily) until they're golden brown, 5 to 7 minutes. Set them aside.

Preheat the oven to 425 degrees F.

Pat the eggplant dry with a paper towel, then toss the cubes with 2 tablespoons of the oil in a large mixing bowl. Spread them out on a baking sheet and roast until they're soft and golden brown,

20 to 25 minutes. (After about 10 minutes, give the eggplant a stir to make sure the cubes are roasting evenly.)

Take the kraut out of the jar with a clean fork, letting any extra brine drain back into it. Roughly chop the kraut, and put it in a small mixing bowl, along with the remaining 1 tablespoon oil, garlic, lemon zest, and lemon juice. Whisk to combine. Pour the kraut mixture over the farro and toss to coat.

Fold the eggplant and basil into the farro and season to taste with salt and pepper if needed. Top with the pine nuts. Serve warm or at room temperature.

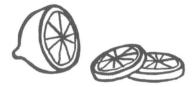

Paprika Potatoes

Smoked paprika, also known as pimentón, *has finally reached mainstream status in the spice world, and not a minute too soon. Made from pimento peppers that have been dried or smoked over a fire, this spice imparts a robust smoky flavor. As a hearty side, this dish pairs well with your favorite sausages, pork loin, or any grilled meat. Leftovers are delicious with eggs in a breakfast burrito or scrambled into a breakfast hash.*

Makes 4 to 6 servings

6 tablespoons extra-virgin olive oil, butter, or coconut oil

1 large or 2 small yellow onions, diced (about 2 cups)

6 medium unpeeled red potatoes, cut into medium dice (about 3 cups)

½ teaspoon paprika

½ teaspoon smoked paprika (*pimentón*)

½ teaspoon salt

1 teaspoon freshly ground black pepper

4 cups stemmed, thinly sliced kale (about ½ pound)

1 cup Caraway Kraut (page 41)

Heat the oil in a large sauté pan over medium heat. Add the onions and sauté until translucent, about 10 minutes. Add the potatoes and sauté, stirring every few minutes, until they're tender, another 15 to 18 minutes. Add the paprika, smoked paprika, salt, and pepper. Sauté until the spices are fragrant, about 1 minute. Add the kale and sauté until it's just wilted but still vibrantly green, 2 to 3 minutes. Remove the pan from the heat and transfer the potato mixture to a large serving bowl.

Take the kraut out of the jar with a clean fork, letting any extra brine drain back into it. Roughly chop the kraut and add it to the potatoes, tossing thoroughly to incorporate.

Serve immediately, while the potatoes are still warm.

> Try soaking cubed potatoes in a bowl of water for an hour to help release the starches, which will help prevent sticking. Drain and lightly dry the potatoes with a towel before cooking.

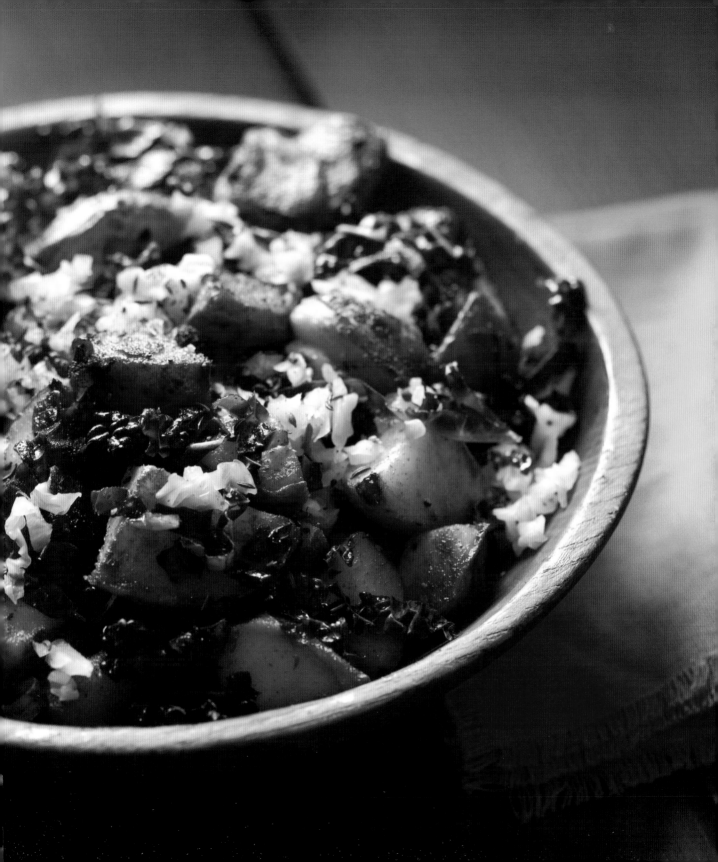

Baked Cortido Polenta

Making polenta from scratch has a bit of a daunting reputation, probably because of all the stirring thought to be involved. Yes, there are recipes that call for stirring so long that your arm tires before the polenta has cooked, but this isn't one of them. You can get away with just giving it an occasional stir, and the result is decadently creamy and much less tiring.

A versatile dish, polenta can be the base for a huge variety of ingredients, including roasted vegetables, meat or tomato sauces, stews, or grilled meats. A one-up on the classic polenta, this recipe is spiced and spiked with a bit of Cortido Kraut and baked into a solid form. That makes it perfect to serve beneath a Bolognese sauce or turn into a pizza-like meal with melted cheese, meats, and veggies on top. Or enjoy it just as it is—delightfully simple, creamy, and satiating.

Makes 6 to 10 servings

2 tablespoons butter

1 small yellow onion, finely diced (about ½ cup)

3 cloves garlic, minced

1 (14-ounce) can diced tomatoes with liquid

2 cups polenta or coarse cornmeal

½ teaspoon salt

1 cup dry white wine

4 cups vegetable or chicken stock

½ cup Cortido Kraut (page 47), plus extra for serving

½ cup grated Parmesan cheese (about 2 ounces) (optional)

Preheat oven to 400 degrees F.

Melt the butter in a large pot over medium heat. Add the onions and sauté until translucent, about 10 minutes. Add the garlic and sauté until golden and fragrant, about 2 minutes. Add the tomatoes with their liquid, polenta, salt, white wine, and vegetable stock, and bring to a boil. Reduce the heat and simmer, stirring every 5 minutes or so until the mixture pulls away from the edges of the pot and all the liquid has been absorbed, 15 to 20 minutes. Remove the pan from the heat.

Take the kraut out of the jar with a clean fork, letting any extra brine drain back into it. Roughly chop the kraut, and add it to the thickened polenta, stirring to incorporate. At this point you can serve or eat the polenta porridge-style if you wish. The following steps transform it into a solid form that can be cut into wedges or squares.

Grease a baking sheet, Pyrex dish, or cast-iron pan—the smaller the pan, the thicker the pieces of polenta will be. Pour the polenta onto the sheet, sprinkle the Parmesan over top, and bake until lightly browned, 20 to 25 minutes.

Let the polenta cool for at least 20 minutes before serving, giving it time to solidify. Slice it into squares or wedges and serve with extra kraut.

Make It Quick & Simple

In a large pot, bring 6 cups of stock or water to a boil. Add 2 cups of polenta in a thin stream, stirring constantly. (This is to avoid lumping.) Cook, stirring frequently, until thick, about 20 minutes. Stir in 2 to 4 tablespoons of butter.

Remove from the heat and serve porridge-style, or pour evenly into a baking dish and let cool in the fridge. With this method, you can slice the polenta into squares and use it as a vehicle for a dip like the Sun-Dried Tomato Tapenade (page 104) or Olive Bean Tapenade (page 97).

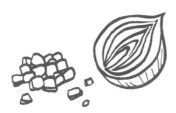

Chickpea Lentil Sauté

A quick and healthy lunch or side dish, this sauté comes together in minutes when you have cooked legumes on hand (see Legumes, page 215, for cooking instructions for both the chickpeas and lentils). Simple, nourishing, and filling, it makes a great accompaniment to grilled chicken or fish, and works well as a base to the Kimchi Red Curry (page 191) in place of rice. It's tasty, filling, and flavorful enough to be a stand-alone meal too.

Makes 4 to 6 servings

2 tablespoons extra-virgin olive oil

2 cups cooked chickpeas, or 1 (15-ounce) can, drained

1 cup cooked lentils (see Legumes, page 215, for cooking instructions)

2 cloves garlic, crushed and minced

1 teaspoon ground turmeric

1 to 2 cups arugula

½ cup Emerald City Kraut (page 49)

⅓ cup crumbled feta cheese (about 1½ ounces)

Salt and freshly ground black pepper

Heat the oil in a large pan over medium-high heat. Add the chickpeas and lentils, and sauté until warm, about 3 minutes. Add the garlic and turmeric and continue to cook, stirring frequently, until they are fragrant, about 1 minute. Remove the pan from the heat.

Stir in the arugula, kraut, and feta just before serving. Season to taste with salt and pepper. Serve warm or at room temperature.

Chapter 10:
Main Meals

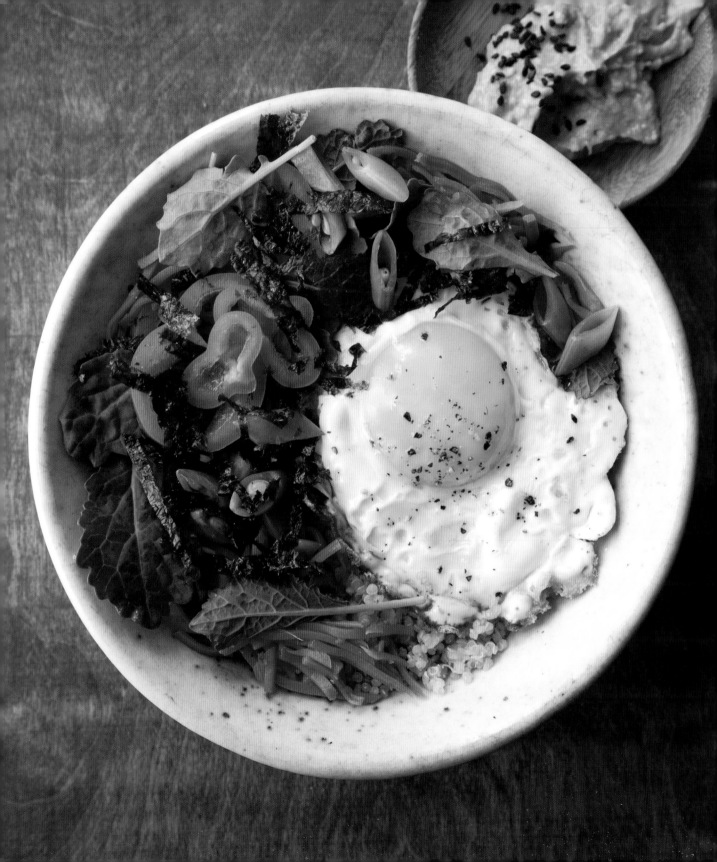

Buddha Bowls with Avocado Sauce

Our Buddha Bowl is a super-nourishing, earthy combination of grains, greens, veggies, and two kinds of ferments—a complete and well-balanced meal in a bowl. This beautifully simple dish is a great way to use up leftover grains and veggies for a healthy dinner or lunch when you're short on time. Cook a big batch of your favorite grain or legume at the beginning of the week and then customize the dish to your liking with fresh or cooked veggies and other goodies all week long.

The recipe calls for Yin Yang Carrots, but any kraut you have on hand will work—better yet, use a combination. Instead of hard-boiled eggs, you could fry up eggs just before you're ready to serve your Buddha Bowl. The avocado sauce is the finishing touch—it makes just about anything taste good—and nicely complements the flavors and textures of the other ingredients.

Divide the spinach among 4 to 6 shallow bowls and top with equal amounts of quinoa and lentils, dividing them among the bowls. Finish each bowl with a few strips of nori, 1 egg, and equal amounts of the fresh veggies. Take the carrots out of the jar with a clean fork, letting any extra brine drain back into it, and divide equally among the bowls.

continued

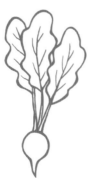

Makes 4 to 6 servings

4 cups spinach or other salad greens (about ½ pound)

4 cups cooked quinoa or brown rice, warm (see Quinoa, page 216, or Rice, page 214, for cooking instructions)

4 cups cooked lentils, warm (see Legumes, page 215, for cooking instructions)

4 sheets nori, cut into thin strips

4 organic, hard-boiled eggs, sliced

2 cups sliced fresh seasonal veggies (such as carrots, avocados, cucumbers, or peppers)

2 to 3 cups Yin Yang Carrots (page 55)

FOR THE SAUCE:

⅓ cup Classic Kraut (page 29)

¼ cup roughly chopped fresh parsley

1 large clove garlic, crushed

1 large avocado, halved, pitted, and peeled

2 tablespoons white miso paste

1 teaspoon Dijon mustard

1 cup water

Salt and freshly ground black pepper

2 tablespoons black sesame seeds, for garnish (optional)

To make the sauce, put all the ingredients except the salt and pepper into a blender or food processor, and blend until smooth. Thin the dressing with additional water if needed, and season to taste with salt and pepper.

Drizzle a few tablespoons of the dressing over each bowl and garnish with the sesame seeds. Serve immediately.

DON'T HEAT YOUR MISO

Often enjoyed as a healing soup for breakfast in the macrobiotic diet or in many Asian cultures, miso has become fairly mainstream in the Western kitchen. While miso can be salty or sweet, light or dark, and mild or rich, it's always best not to heat this tasty paste that is made from fermented soybeans, barley, rice, or rye. High heat can kill the live enzymes and healthy bacteria that are abundant in miso just like our live krauts.

Flank Steak over Spicy Noodles

Rice noodles coated in a creamy coconut sauce and tender pieces of incredibly flavorful flank steak make a killer combination. This dish has it all—robust flavors, crunchy and creamy textures, and plenty of protein. The longer you marinate the steak, the more tasty and tender it will be, so plan a few hours ahead. If you're looking to round out the meal, add as many extra veggies to the noodles as you want; we suggest raw snap peas, steamed asparagus, or grilled eggplant.

For a lighter noodle with different texture, use maifun, *an angel hair–style rice noodle. To make a vegetarian version of this dish, marinate and grill thick slices of eggplant or portabello mushrooms just as you would the steak.*

This dish is great served at room temperature and packs well for potlucks or picnics. Or serve it hot to take the chill off a crisp winter day.

To make the marinade, whisk together the garlic, olive oil, sesame oil, vinegar, brown sugar, and tamari in a small bowl. Put the flank steak in a shallow glass dish or sturdy ziplock bag. Pour the marinade over the steak and cover the dish or seal the bag. Refrigerate for at least 1 hour and up to 8 hours.

Wait until you're ready to grill the steak to cook the noodles. To make the noodles, put them in a large heat-proof bowl. Bring 8 cups of water to a boil, and pour the boiling water over the noodles until they're submerged. Let them sit, stirring every 2 or 3 minutes to keep them from clumping, until they're soft but not mushy, about 10 minutes. Drain the noodles, rinse them under cold water, and put them in a large mixing bowl.

Take the kimchi out of the jar with a clean fork, letting any extra brine drain back into it. Roughly chop the kimchi and add 1½ cups to the noodles, along with the cucumbers, red and yellow bell peppers, green onions, and ½ cup of the cilantro. Toss to combine.

continued

Makes 4 to 6 servings

FOR THE MARINADE:

2 cloves garlic, minced

3 tablespoons extra-virgin olive oil

1 tablespoon sesame oil

3 tablespoons red wine vinegar

2 tablespoons packed brown sugar

⅓ cup tamari

2 pounds flank steak

FOR THE NOODLES:

8 ounces flat rice noodles

2½ cups Firefly Kimchi (page 53), divided

2 large cucumbers, halved, seeded, and thinly sliced crosswise

1 large red bell pepper, cored, seeded, and cut into matchsticks

1 large yellow bell pepper,
cored, seeded, and cut into
matchsticks

6 green onions, chopped,
including the green tops

1 cup chopped fresh cilantro,
divided

FOR THE DRESSING:

Juice of ½ medium lime (about
1 tablespoon)

1 teaspoon Sriracha or your
favorite hot sauce

1 cup coconut milk

1 tablespoon minced fresh
ginger

1 tablespoon fish sauce (aka
nam pla or *nuoc mam*)

3 tablespoons tamari

2 tablespoons sesame oil

4 to 6 lime wedges

¾ cup peanuts or cashews,
roughly chopped

To make the dressing, whisk all of the ingredients in a small bowl until smooth. Set the dressing aside.

Preheat the grill. Remove the steak from the marinade and grill it on one side for 4 to 5 minutes. Flip the steak and grill it for another 4 to 5 minutes, or until it's cooked to your liking. Remove the steak from the grill and let it rest, covered, for about 5 minutes.

While the steak is resting, pour the dressing over the noodles and toss to thoroughly combine. Divide the noodles among the serving plates.

Thinly slice the steak against the grain and at a slight diagonal. (You should end up with long, thin strips.) Lay 4 to 6 strips over each serving of noodles. Top with the remaining 1 cup kimchi and ½ cup cilantro, lime wedges, and peanuts, and serve right away.

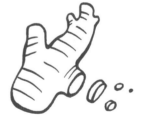

Slow-Roasted Pulled Pork and Kraut

This recipe was created by Suzanne Cameron of Cameron Catering, who generously shared her kitchen with us when Firefly was just getting started. One evening, as we were working late, Suzanne and her kitchen crew returned from an event with leftovers of some of the most incredible pulled pork we had ever tasted. Sweet, salty, spicy, and tender, it went down like candy. With a warning that you pay for flavor with lead time, Suzanne gave us her recipe.

This dish certainly takes some advance planning—the pork takes up to eight hours to brine and then five or more hours to roast—but it's worth every minute. Brining helps keep the meat juicy and tender, but if you don't have time, it will still be delicious. This recipe makes extra rub, so put the leftovers into a jar—it's fantastic on chicken, flank steak, even fried potatoes—and store it for up to six months in the refrigerator.

Serve the pulled pork on buns, over grains, or atop a bed of fresh greens. Try it with a serving of Kimchi Coleslaw (page 120) on the side.

Stir together the salt, maple syrup, and water in a large bowl, and put the pork in it. (Or put the pork in a sturdy, large ziplock bag and pour the brine over it.) Cover the bowl or seal the bag. Make sure the meat is submerged, or flip it every few hours. Refrigerate for 4 to 8 hours.

When you're ready to roast the pork, make the rub by thoroughly mixing all the ingredients in a medium bowl, making sure no clumps of sugar or spices remain.

Preheat the oven to 325 degrees F.

Remove the pork from the marinade, discarding the liquid, and pat it dry. Put the pork in a large roasting pan, fat side up. Generously cover it with the rub (you'll have some left over), and massage the rub into the meat. Cover the pan with aluminum foil and put it in the oven.

Roast until the pork is pull-apart tender, or the internal temperature at the center of the shoulder reads between 200 and 225 degrees F on a meat thermometer. It will take 1 to 1½ hours

continued

Makes 8 to 14 servings

½ cup salt

½ cup maple syrup

2 quarts cold water

1 (5-pound) pork shoulder

FOR THE RUB:

¼ cup packed brown sugar

¼ cup granulated sugar

¼ cup salt

2 tablespoons garlic salt

1 tablespoon onion salt

1½ teaspoons celery salt

¼ cup sweet paprika
(Hungarian preferred)

1 tablespoon chili powder

1 tablespoon freshly ground
black pepper

1½ teaspoons ground sage

½ teaspoon ground allspice

¼ teaspoon cayenne pepper

Pinch of ground cloves

4 to 6 cups Caraway Kraut
(page 41), Ruby Red Kraut
(page 43) (or a mix of both),
or your favorite, for serving

per pound. When it's done, turn off the oven and let the pork rest in the cooling oven for another 30 minutes.

While the pork is still warm, put it on a large cutting board. Peel away the fat from the top surface and discard it. Pull the meat apart using two large forks—it should easily separate into small threads—including the crispier parts that were exposed while roasting.

Serve warm with the kraut.

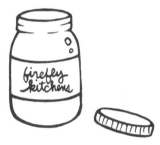

Chicken Satay with Rice Noodles

When we first dreamed up our delicious PB Chi Spread, we incorporated it into as many recipes as we could think of. This dish, with skewered chunks of flavorful chicken, was one of the winners. It's perfectly filling but light, creamy but fresh, and spicy but cooling. Serve it chilled on a hot summer day or warm for a deeply satisfying fall or winter meal. Cilantro, sliced and toasted almonds, and sesame seeds make great garnishes.

Cut the chicken into ½-inch cubes and put them in a medium bowl or sturdy ziplock bag.

To make the marinade, whisk all of the ingredients in a small bowl until smooth. Pour the marinade over the chicken, cover the bowl or seal the plastic bag, and refrigerate for at least 30 minutes and up to 8 hours.

When you're ready to cook the chicken, preheat your barbecue or stovetop grill. Remove the chicken cubes from the marinade and skewer them. Grill the skewers, rotating 45 degrees every 2 to 3 minutes, until all sides have grill marks and the chicken is cooked through, about 8 minutes total.

Meanwhile, put the noodles in a large heatproof bowl. Bring the water to a boil. Pour the boiling water over the noodles until they're submerged, and let them sit, stirring every 2 or 3 minutes to keep them from clumping, until they're soft but not mushy, about 10 minutes. Drain the noodles, rinse them with cold water, and put them in a large mixing bowl.

continued

Makes 4 to 6 servings

4 boneless chicken breasts or about 8 boneless thighs, without skin

FOR THE MARINADE:

2 tablespoons extra-virgin olive oil

Juice of ½ medium lime (about 1 tablespoon)

1 tablespoon apple cider vinegar

1 tablespoon tamari

2 teaspoons packed brown sugar

½ teaspoon ground turmeric

½ teaspoon ground coriander

⅓ teaspoon cayenne pepper

1 tablespoon Sriracha or other hot sauce (optional)

2 tablespoons fish sauce (aka *nam pla* or *nuoc mam*, optional)

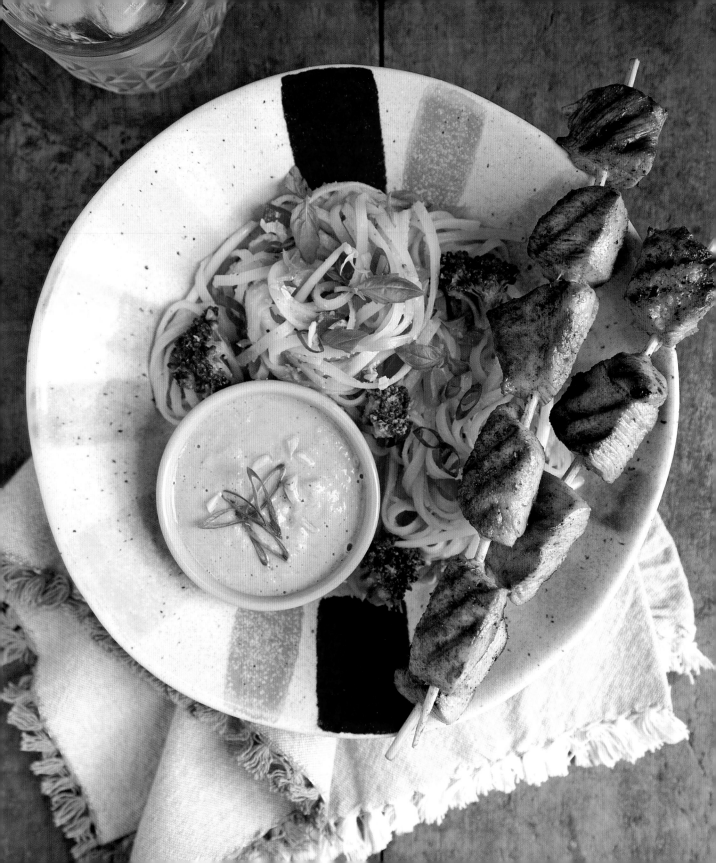

In a small bowl, whisk the spread with the apple cider vinegar and enough water to thin it just a bit. Add the broccoli, green onions, bell pepper, and kimchi to the noodles. Slide the chicken off the skewers and add it to the noodle mixture. Add the thinned spread and toss until well mixed. Garnish with the peanuts, bean sprouts, and basil, and serve immediately.

AMAZING TURMERIC

Turmeric, a member of the ginger family, is well-known for its distinguished taste and color while providing digestive and liver support. *Curicumin*, which is the active ingredient in turmeric, is an antibacterial, antitumor, and anti-inflammatory agent.

10 to 12 skewers, soaked in water if made of wood

12 ounces flat rice noodles

10 cups water

1½ cups PB Chi Spread (page 105)

2 tablespoons apple cider vinegar

2 to 4 tablespoons water

3 cups small broccoli florets, steamed or raw (about ½ pound)

¼ cup sliced green onion, including the green tops

⅓ cup diced red bell pepper

1 cup Firefly Kimchi (page 53)

¼ cup peanuts, chopped, for garnish (optional)

1 cup bean sprouts, for garnish (optional)

¼ cup sliced fresh basil, for garnish (optional)

Black Bean–Sweet Potato Hand Pies

With a delicious, flaky crust wrapped around a tender, earthy, and flavorful filling, these hand pies are perfect little packages of goodness. This recipe is our twist on what's called an empanada in Spanish cooking, a piroshki in Russia, and a calzone in Italy—folding dough around a filling before baking is a traditional technique in cuisines around the world.

This is a fun recipe to make when friends are visiting or kids are ready to help in the kitchen. Rolling the dough, mixing the filling, and making the hand pies goes much faster with a few extra hands. Spice the pies up or add meat, fish, tofu, or seasonal veggies to make it your own.

Makes 12 to 14 hand pies

FOR THE CRUST:

2¼ cups all-purpose flour, plus more for dusting

½ teaspoon salt

½ cup (1 stick) cold, unsalted butter, cut into cubes

1 large organic egg

⅓ cup ice water

1 tablespoon apple cider vinegar or white vinegar

FOR THE FILLING:

½ cup Cortido Kraut (page 47)

2 tablespoons butter or coconut oil

1 large yellow onion, cut into medium dice (about 1⅓ cups)

3 cloves garlic, minced

1 medium jalapeño, seeded and finely diced (about 3 tablespoons)

1 teaspoon ground cumin

1 teaspoon chili powder

1 teaspoon paprika

To make the dough, sift the flour and salt together in a large bowl. Add the butter and blend it into the flour using your fingertips or a pastry blender until the mixture resembles a coarse meal.

In a small bowl, whisk together the egg, water, and vinegar. Add the egg mixture to the flour mixture and mix until the dough begins to clump together. At this point the dough will be a bit stringy and inconsistent (not formed) but that's okay.

Turn the dough out onto a clean, lightly floured work surface. Dust your hands with flour and knead the dough with the heel and palm of your hand until it comes together, adding a few teaspoons of extra flour if the dough sticks to your hands. After kneading for 1 minute or so, the dough should be smooth and hold together in a ball. Pat the ball of dough into a 1-inch-thick round and wrap it tightly with plastic wrap. Refrigerate the dough for at least 1 hour and up to 1 week.

When you're ready to bake the hand pies, remove the dough from the refrigerator and let it come to room temperature, about 30 minutes.

While the dough comes to room temperature, make the filling. Take the kraut out of the jar with a clean fork, letting any extra brine drain back into it. Roughly chop the kraut and set it aside.

Melt the butter in a large sauté pan over medium heat. Add the onion and sauté until translucent, about 10 minutes. Add the garlic and sauté until fragrant, 2 to 3 minutes. Add the jalapeño, cumin, chili powder, paprika, and salt. Sauté, stirring constantly, until the spices release their fragrance, 1 to 2 minutes. Remove the pan from the heat and stir in the kraut, black beans, and sweet potato.

Preheat the oven to 400 degrees F and grease a large baking sheet.

Divide the dough into 10 to 12 pieces. Lightly flour a clean work surface and roll out each piece of dough into a ¼-inch-thick round, about 7 inches in diameter. Scoop about ¼ cup of the filling into the center of each round. Brush the edges of the rounds with a small amount of the egg whites. Fold the dough over the filling, creating a half-moon shape, and press the edges together to seal, crimping them together with a fork for a little frill if you want. Brush the top of each pie with egg white and cut a small slit for steam to escape. Put the pies on the prepared baking sheet and bake until golden brown, 15 to 18 minutes.

While the pies are baking, make the dipping sauce. Take the kraut out of the jar using a clean fork, letting any extra brine drain back into it, and mince the kraut. Put the kraut, sour cream, hot sauce, and cilantro in a blender or food processor. Whirl until smooth and season to taste with salt and pepper.

When the hand pies are done, transfer them to a serving platter. Serve piping hot with the dipping sauce on the side or drizzled over the top of the pies.

2 teaspoons salt

2 cups cooked black beans, or 1 (15-ounce) can, drained (see Legumes, page 215, for cooking instructions)

1½ cups cooked sweet potato or yam, skin removed and roughly mashed (about 1 pound sweet potatoes)

2 egg whites, lightly whisked, for brushing the pies before baking

FOR THE DIPPING SAUCE:

¾ cup Cortido Kraut (page 47)

1 cup sour cream or plain yogurt

½ to 1 teaspoon hot sauce of your choice

4 tablespoons fresh cilantro, chopped

Salt and freshly ground black pepper

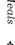

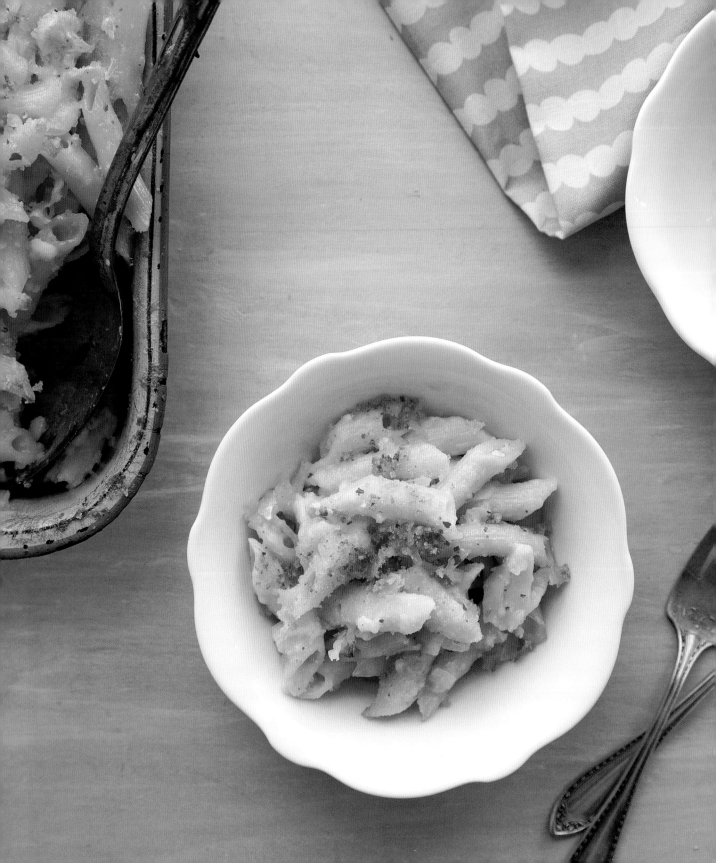

Kimchi'd Mac and Cheese

This recipe transforms that classic comfort food, mac and cheese, into a slightly spicy, nourishing delicacy for grown-ups. As it cooks, the pieces of cauliflower break down into the cheesy sauce, creating an earthy, rich, and intensely creamy flavor. Serve this dish with a big bowl of lightly dressed greens, and you've got a satisfying meal.

Preheat the oven to 350 degrees F and grease a 13-by-9-inch baking pan.

Put the water and salt in a large pot, and bring it to a boil. Add the penne and cook, following the package directions, until it's tender yet firm to the bite. Drain the pasta well. Return it to the pot (off the heat) and toss it with the oil.

Melt the butter over medium heat in a medium sauté pan. Add the onion and sauté until translucent, about 10 minutes. Sprinkle the flour over the onions and stir, cooking for another minute. Slowly add the milk, stirring constantly, until the mixture comes to a simmer. Add both cheeses, stirring until melted. Remove the pan from the heat and pour the mixture over the cooked pasta. Mix in the cauliflower.

Take the kimchi out of the jar with a clean fork, letting any extra brine drain back into it. Roughly chop the kimchi and mix it into the pasta. Season to taste with salt and pepper.

Spread the pasta mixture evenly in the prepared pan. Top with the bread crumbs, and bake until bubbly and brown, 30 to 35 minutes.

Serve piping hot with an additional dollop of kimchi.

Make It Quick & Simple

Make your favorite quick macaroni and cheese—homemade or boxed. When it's off the heat, stir in a cup of chopped Firefly Kimchi.

Makes 4 to 6 servings

6 quarts water

1 tablespoon salt

1 pound penne pasta

1 tablespoon extra-virgin olive oil

¼ cup unsalted butter (½ stick)

1 medium onion, diced

¼ cup unbleached, all-purpose flour

3 cups milk

4 cups shredded sharp white cheddar cheese (1 pound)

1½ cups shredded Swiss cheese (about 6 ounces)

4 cups finely chopped cauliflower (about 1 medium cauliflower)

1½ cups Firefly Kimchi (page 53), plus extra for garnish

Salt and freshly ground black pepper

1 cup fresh bread crumbs

Emerald City Meatloaf

While meatloaf is often regarded as a bit old-school, we believe it deserves a space in every meat-eater's repertoire. A comforting meatloaf can quell the hunger of a crowd and is deeply flavorful and moist. It has just enough fat to keep it from crumbling and seal in flavor without being bathed in grease. It's simple and filling, and results in some of the best sandwich-making leftovers (Richard has fond memories of the next-day sandwiches his father would make—toast with thick slices of meatloaf and lots of black pepper).

When you're considering which vegetables to use, you might include in your mix carrots, onions, mushrooms, bell peppers, garlic, or whatever you have on hand and appeals to your taste buds.

Thickly slice the meatloaf to serve a few hungry souls, or slice it thinner and serve it with a side of Caraway-Kale-Cauliflower Fluff (page 151) and a heaping bowl of Krauty Kale Caesar (page 116) to feed a crowd. Of course, we always serve it with a big bowl of extra kraut to top it off. Any kraut you like would be a great side for this meatloaf.

Makes 6 to 8 servings

- 1 tablespoon olive or coconut oil
- 1 cup minced vegetables of your choice
- 1 tablespoon minced fresh parsley
- 1 pound lean ground beef
- 1 pound ground pork
- 1 large organic egg
- ¼ cup fresh bread crumbs
- 1 tablespoon Worcestershire sauce
- ½ cup plus 1 teaspoon steak sauce

Preheat the oven to 350 degrees F and grease an 8-by-4-inch loaf pan.

Heat the oil in a large sauté pan over medium heat. Add the vegetables and parsley and sauté until they just begin to soften and lose their moisture, 3 to 4 minutes. Remove the pan from the heat and let the vegetables cool.

Combine the ground beef, pork, egg, bread crumbs, Worcestershire sauce, and steak sauce in a large bowl. Take the kraut out of the jar with a clean fork, letting any extra brine drain back into it. Roughly chop the kraut and add it to the meat mixture. Add the cooled veggies, salt, and pepper, and mix everything together until well incorporated.

Press the meatloaf evenly into the prepared pan. Bake until a meat thermometer inserted in the middle of the loaf reads 160 degrees F, 45 to 50 minutes. Remove the pan from the oven and carefully pour off any excess fat. Let the meatloaf cool slightly.

To make the sauce, take the kraut out of the jar using a clean fork, letting any extra brine drain back into it, then roughly chop the kraut. Combine the kraut, ketchup, Worcestershire sauce, and steak sauce in a blender or food processor, and whirl until smooth. Spread the sauce over the loaf while it's still hot, so that it gently warms the sauce. Slice the meatloaf to your desired thickness and serve with an extra spoonful of kraut on the side.

¼ cup Emerald City Kraut (page 49)

Pinch of salt and freshly ground black pepper

FOR THE SAUCE:

1 cup Classic Kraut (page 29) or Caraway Kraut (page 41), plus more for serving (optional)

½ cup ketchup

2 teaspoons Worcestershire sauce

2 teaspoons steak sauce (optional)

Pea and Prosciutto Risotto

When it comes to risotto, patience is the name of the game. Yes, stirring a pot of rice and broth for twenty minutes can seem tedious, but the finished product is truly worth it—the more you stir, the creamier it gets, and the more complex and melded the flavors become. Even though it has no butter or cheese, this risotto is amazingly rich and velvety. Classic Kraut balances the creaminess with a pop of flavor. The risotto melts in your mouth like savory candy.

Leftovers can be formed into patties and fried, or pan-seared until golden brown, and served as a light meal or appetizer. Top risotto cakes with Sun-Dried Tomato Tapenade (page 104), Smoked Salmon Mousse (page 96), or just about any other sauce or spread.

Makes 6 to 8 servings

⅓ cup plus 1 tablespoon extra-virgin olive oil, divided

1 large yellow onion, chopped

4 cloves garlic, chopped

4 cups arborio rice

2 quarts chicken or vegetable stock, divided

1 cup white wine, divided

2 cups frozen peas

1¼ cups Classic Kraut (page 29), divided

4 ounces prosciutto, diced

½ cup chopped fresh parsley (optional)

Heat ½ cup of the oil in a medium, heavy-bottomed pot over medium heat. Add the onions and sauté until translucent, about 10 minutes. Add the garlic and sauté until fragrant, 2 to 3 minutes.

Add the rice and cook, stirring frequently, until it just begins to stick to the bottom of the pan, 4 to 5 minutes. Add ½ cup of the chicken stock and 2 tablespoons of the wine, stirring until the liquid is absorbed. Repeat this process, adding the liquid and stirring until it's absorbed, until you've used all the stock and wine. Add the peas during the last 5 minutes of cooking and stir to combine, cooking until the peas are warm and all the liquid has been absorbed.

Take the kraut out of the jar with a clean fork, letting any extra brine drain back into it. Roughly chop the kraut.

Heat the remaining 1 tablespoon of oil in a small sauté pan over medium heat. Add ¼ cup of the chopped kraut and the prosciutto, and sauté until the prosciutto just begins to brown, about 5 minutes. Remove the pan from the heat and stir its contents into the risotto.

Portion the risotto into serving bowls. Distribute the remaining 1 cup kraut evenly over each serving. Garnish with the parsley and serve immediately.

Halibut with Avocado Butter

Years have passed since Julie's wedding at Ross Lake Resort in Rockport, Washington, yet friends still remember the fish she served. Her uncle, Skip Bolton, a passionate fisherman, generously provided 150 pounds of halibut, which he prepared with an incredibly scrumptious avocado butter.

Still enamored with this meal, Julie discovered that Classic Kraut (page 29) added a fresh new dimension to the avocado butter. Pair the halibut with Scarlet Millet (page 150) and Emerald City Salad (page 115) for a well-rounded and festive dinner.

To make the marinade, put the halibut in a large dish or ziplock bag. In a medium bowl, whisk together the oil, tamari, mustard, lemon zest, lemon juice, and garlic. Pour the marinade over the fish and cover the dish or seal the bag. Refrigerate for at least 30 minutes or up to 2 hours. Flip the fish every 30 minutes so it's evenly marinated on both sides.

When you're ready to bake the fish, preheat the oven to 400 degrees F and grease a heatproof baking dish.

Remove the halibut from the marinade, discarding the liquid, and put it into the prepared baking dish. Bake the halibut until it visibly begins to flake apart in the middle, or an instant-read thermometer registers a temperature of 145 degrees F when inserted into the thickest part of the fillet, 12 to 18 minutes, depending on the thickness. After removing it from the oven, tent the baking dish with aluminum foil. Let the halibut rest for 5 minutes.

While the halibut rests, make the avocado butter. Put the kraut, butter, and avocado in a food processor and whirl until smooth. Add the lemon juice, parsley, and garlic, and blend until creamy. Season to taste with salt and pepper.

Serve the halibut immediately, either whole on a large platter with the avocado butter evenly spread on top, or sliced into individual portions, topping each with 2 to 3 tablespoons of the butter.

Makes 4 servings

FOR THE MARINADE:

One 1½-pound halibut fillet

½ cup extra-virgin olive oil

⅓ cup tamari

2 teaspoons Dijon mustard

1 teaspoon lemon zest

¼ teaspoon freshly squeezed lemon juice

1 clove garlic, minced

FOR THE AVOCADO BUTTER:

½ cup Classic Kraut (page 29), finely minced

½ cup (1 stick) butter, softened

1 avocado (the bigger the better), halved, pitted, peeled, and cut into chunks

2 tablespoons freshly squeezed lemon juice

2 tablespoons roughly chopped fresh parsley

2 cloves garlic, minced

Salt and freshly ground black pepper

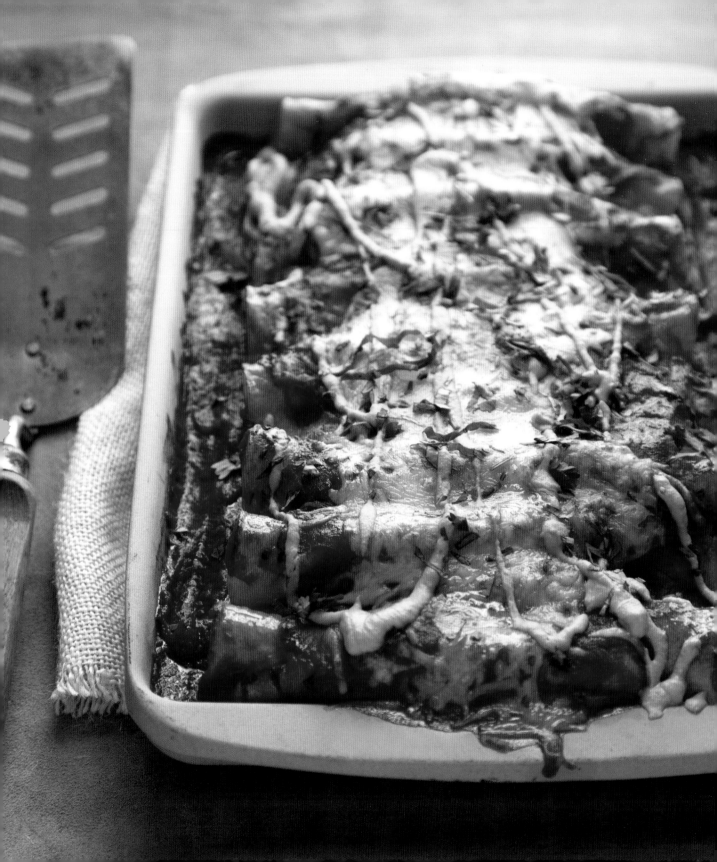

Cortido Enchiladas

These enchiladas are not too cheesy, and they're rich with nourishing greens—the kale adds a hearty dose of fiber, antioxidants, and chlorophyll—making for a lighter recipe than most. If you don't have Cortido Kraut on hand, make the sauce instead with Classic Kraut (page 29), adding a thinly sliced green onion and a pinch of oregano. Play around with the filling ingredients to make this dish your own. We love adding shredded chicken, bell peppers, roasted tomatoes, and zucchini.

Preheat the oven to 350 degrees F and lightly grease a 9-by-13-inch baking dish.

Melt 2 tablespoons of the butter in a large sauté pan over medium heat. Add the onions and sauté until translucent, about 10 minutes. Add the kale, garlic, cumin, salt, and pepper, along with the remaining 2 tablespoons butter, and sauté until the greens are wilted, about 3 minutes.

Remove the pan from the heat, put the kale mixture into a medium bowl, and stir in the beans. When it's cool, mix in 1½ cups of the cheese.

In the same pan, combine the enchilada sauce, tomatoes, and chili powder. Simmer until the flavors meld, about 5 minutes. Spread about ½ cup of the sauce in the prepared baking dish.

Put a tortilla on a clean work surface, spoon about ⅓ cup of the kale mixture into the center, and top with 1 tablespoon of the sauce. Roll up each tortilla around the mixture to form a log and lay it, seam side down, in the baking dish. Repeat until all the tortillas have been filled and are lined up next to one another in the dish. Pour the remaining red sauce over the tortillas. Spread the sauce evenly, making sure you coat all the tortilla edges.

continued

Makes 6 to 8 servings

¼ cup (½ stick) butter or extra-virgin olive oil, divided

1 large onion, diced

5 cups stemmed, thin sliced kale or chard (about ¾ pound)

4 cloves smashed garlic, roughly chopped

1 teaspoon ground cumin

1 teaspoon salt

½ teaspoon freshly ground black pepper

1½ cups cooked black beans, or 1 (15-ounce) can (see Legumes, page 215, for cooking instructions)

2 cups (½ pound) grated sharp white cheddar cheese, divided

1 (14-ounce) can enchilada sauce

1 (14-ounce) can diced tomatoes

1 teaspoon chili powder

Ten 10-inch flour or corn tortillas

FOR THE SAUCE:

1 cup Cortido Kraut (page 47)

½ cup loosely packed fresh cilantro

⅓ cup raw pumpkin seeds

⅓ cup sour cream

¼ cup shredded sharp cheddar or Cotija cheese (optional)

Salt and freshly ground black pepper

Cover the dish with foil and bake for 20 minutes. Remove the foil, sprinkle the remaining ½ cup cheddar on top, and bake, uncovered, until the cheese is melted and bubbly, another 10 to 15 minutes.

While the enchiladas are baking, make the sauce. Take the kraut out of the jar using a clean fork, letting any extra brine drain back into the jar. Combine all the ingredients except for the salt and pepper in a blender or food processor, and whirl until smooth. Season to taste with salt and pepper. Thin with a splash of brine or water if needed.

Serve the enchiladas hot with the sauce drizzled on top.

Shrimp and Kimchi Fried Rice

This is a great way to use leftover rice and put together a quick, healthy dinner in less than twenty minutes. Throw in as few or as many veggies as you like, and add meat, fish, or tofu—whatever you have on hand. Snap peas, broccoli florets, napa cabbage, bok choy, tofu, chicken, and beef all work well. While the recipe calls for short-grain brown rice, any leftover rice will work. This is a recipe that's easy to double to feed a crowd. Leave out the shrimp, and it makes a tasty breakfast.

Whisk together the chili garlic sauce, fish sauce, and tamari in a small bowl and set it aside.

Heat 1 tablespoon of the coconut oil in a large sauté pan over medium-high heat. When the oil is hot, add the shrimp and cook, stirring frequently, until pink, 2 to 4 minutes, depending on the size of the shrimp. Remove the shrimp from the pan and set it aside.

Add the remaining 2 tablespoons coconut oil to the pan and lower the heat to medium. Add the onion and sauté until translucent, about 10 minutes. Add the jalapeño and garlic and sauté until fragrant, 2 to 3 minutes. Add the rice and the sauce mixture, and cook, stirring frequently, for 2 to 3 minutes until the rice is warmed through.

Make a space in the center of the pan by pushing its contents toward the edges. Add the eggs and cook, stirring frequently, until they begin to scramble, about 2 minutes. Mix the eggs with the rest of the pan's ingredients and cook, stirring frequently, for 1 to 2 more minutes.

Add the peas and shrimp and cook until the peas are heated through, 2 to 3 minutes. Transfer the fried rice to a serving bowl. Take the kimchi out of the jar using a clean fork, letting any extra brine drain back into it, then chop the kimchi. Top with the green onions and kimchi, and serve immediately.

Makes 4 to 6 servings

- 1 tablespoon chili garlic sauce
- 1 tablespoon fish sauce (aka *nam pla* or *nuoc mam*)
- 2 tablespoons tamari
- 3 tablespoons coconut oil, divided
- ½ pound peeled whole medium shrimp, rinsed and drained
- 1 small yellow onion, diced (about 1 cup)
- 1 medium jalapeño, finely chopped (about 3 tablespoons)
- 3 cloves garlic, minced
- 2 cups cooked short-grain brown rice (see Rice, page 214, for cooking instructions)
- 2 large organic eggs, beaten
- 2 cups frozen or fresh peas
- 1 cup Firefly Kimchi (page 53)
- 3 green onions, diced, including the green tops

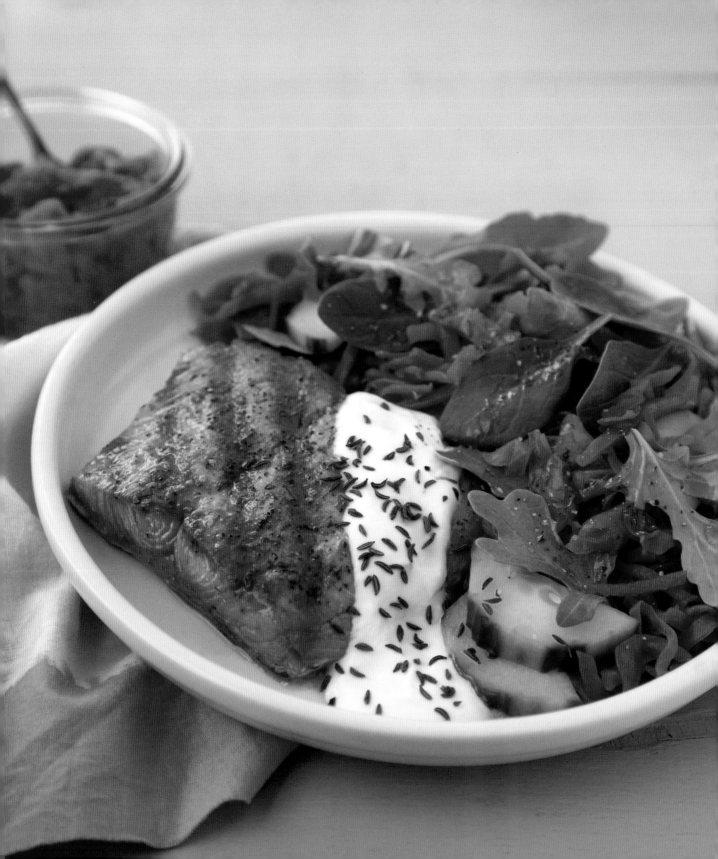

Salmon with Caraway Cream

We're so fortunate in the Pacific Northwest to have access to an abundance of fresh salmon, and we love to experiment with creative ways to prepare it. In other parts of the country, look for frozen salmon, which is often just as good—sometimes better—than what you can buy fresh. We've found that the earthy flavor of caraway seed pairs well with salmon. And in this recipe we give you two ways to cook the fish: grilled or baked.

This attractive dish is perfect for a casual dinner party, served alongside the Caraway-Kale-Cauliflower Fluff (page 151) and roasted asparagus or brussels sprouts. When plating, nestle the salmon alongside the greens or use the greens as a bed and lay the salmon on top. The caraway cream makes a great dressing for the greens as well, so make sure to drizzle it over the entire dish.

Preheat the oven to 400 degrees F or, if you're using a grill, preheat it and carefully oil the hot grates to help keep the fish from sticking.

Let the salmon sit at room temperature for about 15 minutes, and pat it dry with paper towels. Rub 2 tablespoons of the oil and the salt and pepper over the salmon.

IF YOU'RE GRILLING THE SALMON, put the fillet, skin side up, on the hot grill and cook for 5 to 7 minutes. Using a large metal spatula, flip the salmon, keeping the skin intact, and cook for 4 to 6 more minutes. (If the fillet is less than 1 inch thick, it will take 8 to 10 minutes total; if it's between 1 and 2 inches thick, it will take a little longer, 12 to 14 minutes.) When both sides have been seared, gently press your finger or the handle of a knife into the fleshy side of the salmon; if it starts to flake apart, it's done. Take the salmon off the grill and let it rest for about 5 minutes.

IF YOU'RE BAKING THE SALMON, put the fillet, skin side down, on an oiled baking sheet. Bake for about 10 minutes per inch of thickness. At the 8-minute mark, gently press your finger or the handle of a knife into the fleshy side of the salmon; if it starts

continued

Makes 4 to 6 servings

1 (2-pound) salmon fillet

3 tablespoons extra-virgin olive oil, divided

1 teaspoon salt

¼ teaspoon freshly ground black pepper

1 cup Ruby Red Kraut (page 43)

8 cups loosely packed salad greens (about 12 ounces)

1 medium cucumber, peeled and thinly sliced (optional)

FOR THE CARAWAY CREAM:

1 teaspoon caraway seeds

1 cup sour cream, Greek yogurt, or crème fraîche

1½ tablespoons Dijon mustard

1 tablespoon freshly squeezed lemon juice

1 teaspoon lemon zest

1 teaspoon sugar (optional)

1 to 3 tablespoons water

Salt and freshly ground black pepper

to flake apart, it's done. If not, continue to bake and check every 2 minutes, being careful not to overcook it. Transfer the salmon to a plate and let it rest for about 5 minutes.

To make the cream, first crush the caraway seeds using a mortar and pestle, rolling pin, or clean coffee grinder. Break them down, but don't crush them to a powder.

Put the seeds, along with the sour cream, mustard, lemon juice, lemon zest, sugar, and 1 tablespoon water, in a small bowl. Whisk to thoroughly combine, thinning with more water until you get the consistency you like. Season to taste with salt and pepper, and set the cream aside.

Take the kraut out of the jar with a clean fork, letting any extra brine drain back into it. Roughly chop the kraut and put it in a large mixing bowl with the greens, cucumber, and the remaining 1 tablespoon oil. Gently toss to combine.

Cut the salmon into 4 to 6 equal pieces. Evenly divide the greens among 4 to 6 plates. Place a salmon piece next to or on top of the greens on each plate. Drizzle each serving with the cream and serve immediately.

Kimchi Red Curry

The spicy and stimulating flavors of Firefly Kimchi balance the heat of this red curry, while the creamy coconut milk and hint of lime provide calming and cool notes.

In a pinch, you can top any takeout curry with a generous dollop of kimchi to brighten its flavors, but when you have the time, give this recipe a try. The benefits of homemade curry are enormous: you'll have fresher vegetables, more vibrant flavors, and your preferred ingredients: make it as spicy, veggie-packed, gingery, creamy, or mild as you like. Serve this dish family-style.

Heat the oil in a large pot over medium heat. Sauté the chicken, stirring occasionally, until the cubes are slightly browned, about 5 minutes. Add the curry paste, fish sauce, chili sauce, and ginger, and sauté for 1 minute. Add the carrots, green beans, chicken stock, and coconut milk, and bring to a boil. Turn the heat down to low and simmer for 5 more minutes. Remove the pot from the heat and let the curry cool slightly. Stir in the lime juice.

Put the curry and rice in separate serving bowls and put the garnishes—the kimchi, basil, sprouts, and cashews—in smaller bowls, letting your guests serve themselves.

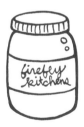

Makes 4 to 6 servings

2 tablespoons coconut oil

2 boneless, skinless chicken breasts (about 1 pound), cut into ½-inch cubes

2 tablespoons red curry paste

1 tablespoon fish sauce (aka *nam pla* or *nuoc mam*)

1 tablespoon chili garlic sauce

1 tablespoon minced fresh ginger

2 large carrots, thinly sliced or cut into matchsticks

¾ pound green beans, tips removed and cut into 1-inch pieces

1 cup chicken stock

1½ cups coconut milk

Juice of 1 medium lime (about 2 tablespoons)

4 cups cooked brown rice (see Rice, page 214, for cooking instructions)

1 cup Firefly Kimchi (page 53)

½ cup chopped fresh basil

½ cup bean sprouts (optional)

½ cup cashews, chopped (optional)

Sun-Dried Tomato Linguine

This is a hearty and easy dinner to prepare, especially if you make the Sun-Dried Tomato-Tapenade ahead of time. Boost the health benefits and tummy-filling factor of this dish by tossing in lots of extra veggies, such as cauliflower, mushrooms, peas, or whatever's in season. You can also transform it into a cold pasta salad by using a bowtie- or pinwheel-shaped pasta and letting it cool before serving. The optional heavy cream makes a rich sauce, but it's delicious any way you choose to make it. Gluten-free pastas work splendidly with this recipe.

Added at the end to preserve the delicate probiotics and digestive enzymes, the fresh kraut adds bright flavor.

Makes 4 to 6 servings

2 cups Sun-Dried Tomato Tapenade (page 104)

½ cup heavy cream (optional)

6 quarts water

1 tablespoon salt

1 pound linguine

1 tablespoon butter or extra-virgin olive oil

1 medium yellow onion, diced (about 2 cups)

2 zucchini (about ½ pound), halved lengthwise and cut into ¼-inch-thick pieces

1 cup Classic Kraut (page 29)

Salt and freshly ground black pepper

4 to 6 tablespoons chopped fresh parsley

½ cup pine nuts

½ cup grated Parmesan cheese (about 2 ounces)

Put the tapenade in a medium bowl, stir in the heavy cream, and set it aside.

Put the water and salt in a large pot, and bring it to a boil. Add the linguine and cook, following the package directions, until it's tender yet firm to the bite. Drain the linguine, reserving about 1 cup of the pasta water for thinning the sauce if needed later on. Put the pasta in a large bowl.

Melt the butter in a large sauté pan over medium heat. Add the onion and sauté for 7 minutes. Add the zucchini and sauté, stirring frequently, until the onions are translucent and the zucchini are soft, 3 to 5 minutes. Add the vegetables to the pasta.

Take the kraut out of the jar using a clean fork, letting any extra brine drain back into it, then chop the kraut. Whirl the kraut in a blender or food processor until it's the consistency of applesauce. Pour the blended kraut and the prepared tapenade over the pasta and toss to thoroughly combine. If the pasta clumps together, add the reserved pasta water, 1 tablespoon at a time, to loosen it up. Season to taste with salt and pepper.

Sprinkle the parsley, pine nuts, and Parmesan over the pasta, and serve immediately.

Chapter 11:
On the Sweet Side

Lemony Cream Delight

We mix sweet, zesty lemon curd with tangy kraut and cream cheese to create an incredibly vibrant but not-too-sweet cream that's perfect for piping into tart shells, spreading between shortbread cookies, frosting your favorite cake, icing a cupcake (or muffin), or using as a sweet dip for fresh fruit. Layer it with fresh berries and crumbled cookies in a big glass bowl to create a beautiful trifle—or, of course, you could just eat it straight from the bowl.

Makes about 2 cups

2 tablespoons butter, at room temperature

Zest of 1 medium lemon (about 1 tablespoon)

⅓ cup sugar

1 large organic egg, at room temperature

Juice from 1 medium lemon (about 3 tablespoons)

Pinch of salt

⅓ cup Classic Kraut (page 29), drained

6 ounces cream cheese, at room temperature

1 tablespoon shredded unsweetened coconut (optional)

In a medium bowl, using an electric mixer or by hand, beat the butter until smooth. Add the lemon zest and sugar and mix until they're well combined. Add the egg, beating until smooth. Add the lemon juice and salt, and beat until smooth.

Put the lemon mixture into a small heavy-bottomed saucepan and cook for 6 to 8 minutes over low heat, stirring constantly. It will start to thicken and take on a deeper yellow color. Take care not to let it boil, or it will curdle. The curd is done when it has thickened and coats a spoon, or when it reads 170 degrees F on an instant-read thermometer. Set it aside to cool. The curd can be covered and refrigerated at this point for up to a week before making the cream.

Take the kraut out of the jar with a clean fork, letting any extra brine drain back into the jar. Mince the kraut finely and squeeze out any extra brine.

When the curd is cool, use an electric mixer or food processor to mix in the kraut and cream cheese until smooth. Fold in the coconut until just combined. Serve right away or refrigerate for up to 3 days.

Make It Quick & Simple

Instead of making the lemon curd, mix ½ cup store-bought lemon curd with the rest of the ingredients. You may want to add a teaspoon of lemon zest to brighten up the end result.

Spiced Roulade with Orange Cream Filling

We put Joey Goeller, a talented baker at Seattle's Cameron Catering, to the challenge of making a spiced rolled cake to hold our orange cream filling. Not only was he successful, but he taught us the secret to this type of cake: thoroughly whipping the egg yolks before adding anything else to the batter, which gives the cake an airy, spongy texture. This is key to making a roulade, which requires a thin cake that's soft and flexible enough to roll up into a log around a creamy filling. When you slice the cake, you'll see festive spirals of cake and filling. His other words of wisdom: have your ingredients at room temperature, measure carefully, don't overmix, and don't overbake.

Add another dimension to this recipe by mixing finely diced candied ginger into the cream or layering sliced strawberries between the cake and cream before rolling it up. There might be more cream here than you need, but you'll know what to do with it.

This cake is best served right away; if you wait too long, it will absorb the cream and lose its light and fluffy texture.

Preheat the oven to 350 degrees F.

Grease a 10-by-15-inch jelly roll pan. Line the bottom of the pan with parchment paper, leaving 3 inches of the parchment hanging over the long side of the pan. (The overhang will give you something to grab when you roll up the cake.) Grease the parchment paper and lightly dust it with all-purpose flour.

Carefully separate the egg yolks from the whites, reserving the whites in a medium bowl. (Make sure there are no specks of yolk in the whites. Even a speck of yolk will keep the whites from expanding to their full volume when you whip them.) Whisk the egg yolks in a large bowl until pale yellow and creamy, about 3 minutes. Whisk in the molasses and melted butter.

continued

Makes 6 to 8 servings

3 organic eggs, at room temperature

½ cup molasses

2 tablespoons butter, melted

1 cup all-purpose flour, plus extra for dusting the pan

¼ teaspoon baking soda

½ teaspoon ground ginger

½ teaspoon ground cinnamon

¼ teaspoon salt

½ cup granulated sugar

Confectioners' sugar, for dusting the cake

FOR THE ORANGE CREAM FILLING:

½ cup Classic Kraut (page 29)

1 pint heavy cream

¼ cup confectioners' sugar

2 tablespoons orange zest

3 tablespoons freshly squeezed orange juice

1 teaspoon vanilla extract

½ cup vanilla yogurt (optional)

In a small bowl, sift together the flour, baking soda, ginger, cinnamon, and salt. Add the dry ingredients to the yolk mixture in two batches, stirring until smooth after each addition and being careful not to overmix.

Using an electric mixer or a whisk, whip the reserved egg whites until frothy. Continue to beat and add the sugar, 1 tablespoon at a time, until the egg whites form stiff, glossy peaks. Using a large spoon or spatula, gently fold a third of the egg whites at a time into the yolk mixture. (You're trying to fully combine them without losing the fluffiness of the whites.) Evenly spread the batter in the prepared pan.

Bake the cake until it feels spongy and springs back to the touch, 7 to 8 minutes.

When you remove the cake from the oven, dust it with a little confectioners' sugar, then put the still-hot cake in its pan on the counter with the excess parchment facing away from you. Lay a dry towel or cloth over the top of the cake and gently pull the parchment flap up and toward you, rolling the cake around the towel. Continue rolling, letting the parchment paper fall away from the cake, until the cake is completely rolled up around the towel. Set the cake seam side down and let it cool completely. (If you accidentally bake the cake too long and it cracks as you roll it, don't worry! When you put the filling in, the cream will fill in the cracks and the cake will be just as delicious.)

While the cake is cooling, make the filling. Take the kraut out of the jar with a clean fork, letting any extra brine drain back into it. Finely mince the kraut.

In a medium bowl, using an electric mixer or a whisk, whip the cream, confectioners' sugar, orange zest, orange juice, and vanilla until the mixture forms stiff peaks. Fold in the minced kraut and yogurt until well mixed.

When the cake is cool and just before you are ready to serve it, carefully unroll it and remove the towel. Spread the filling evenly over the cake and immediately roll it back up. (If you won't be serving the cake right away, leave it rolled up, unfrosted, around the towel at room temperature for no longer than 3 hours—if you wait longer, you run the risk of the cake cracking as it dries out, so keep the cream in the refrigerator.)

To serve, place the cake seam side down on a serving platter and dust it again with confectioners' sugar. Slice it into rounds about 2 inches thick. The resulting slices should look like pinwheels of cake and frosting. Serve immediately.

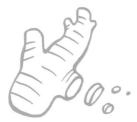

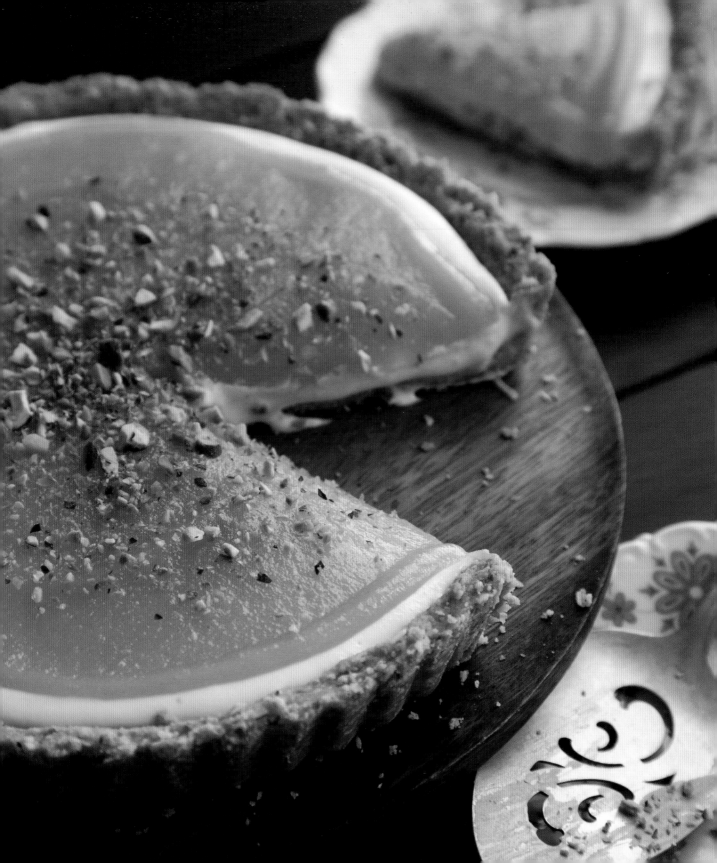

Apricot Goat Cheese Tart

The flavors in this tart are decadent and complex, so it makes a great dessert for any special occasion. The sweet, cookie-like almond crust meets the creamy tart filling to create a not-overly-sweet but definitely indulgent treat.

Preheat the oven to 350 degrees F.

To make the crust, in a small bowl, thoroughly mix the brown sugar, flour, and salt.

Put the almonds and oats in the bowl of a food processor and pulse until finely ground. Add the butter and pulse for another 30 seconds. Add the vanilla and almond extracts and pulse until combined. Add the dry ingredients and pulse until you get a fine, crumbly texture.

Press the mixture into a 9-inch tart pan, evenly distributing it across the bottom and up the sides of the pan. Bake until light golden brown, 12 to 15 minutes. Set the crust aside to cool.

To make the filling, in a medium bowl, using an electric mixer, combine the cream cheese, goat cheese, and yogurt until well blended (or add the ingredients to the bowl of a food processor and pulse until blended). Add the lemon juice and confectioners' sugar and mix until smooth.

Take the kraut out of the jar with a clean fork, letting any extra brine drain back into it. Mince the kraut, squeeze any excess brine out of it, and mix it into the cream filling until thoroughly combined.

continued

Makes one 9-inch tart

FOR THE CRUST:

½ cup packed brown sugar

½ cup unbleached, all-purpose flour

¼ teaspoon salt

½ cup sliced almonds

¼ cup rolled oats

6 tablespoons butter or coconut oil

¼ teaspoon vanilla extract

¼ teaspoon almond extract

FOR THE FILLING:

12 ounces cream cheese, softened

4 ounces goat cheese, softened

⅓ cup Greek yogurt

1 tablespoon freshly squeezed lemon juice

¼ cup confectioners' sugar

⅓ cup Classic Kraut (page 29)

FOR THE APRICOT TOPPING:

½ cup dried apricots, chopped

½ cup water

½ cup Classic Kraut (page 29)

½ cup apricot preserves

½ cup finely chopped pistachios

Pour the filling into the cooled crust, spreading it evenly. Refrigerate until the filling is firm, at least 1 hour.

While the tart filling is chilling, make the apricot topping. Put the apricots in a small heat-resistant glass or ceramic bowl. Bring the water to a boil and pour it over the apricots. Let the apricots sit until they're soft, about 20 minutes. (You can do this step up to 8 hours in advance and leave the apricots sitting in the water, covered, at room temperature.)

Take the kraut out of the jar with a clean fork, letting any extra brine drain back into it, and mince the kraut. Put the apricots, their soaking water, kraut, and preserves into a blender or food processor. Blend until the mixture is completely smooth and set aside to cool.

When the cream filling is firm and the apricot topping is cool, spread the apricot mixture evenly over the top of the tart. Sprinkle the pistachios over the top.

Slice the tart into small wedges and serve immediately, or chill until 30 minutes before serving.

> **CONVERT A DESSERT INTO AN APPETIZER**
>
> For a fantastic appetizer, make the cream cheese filling without the sugar and with a little extra kraut, and serve it with crackers. Or heat up a round of Brie, spread it with the apricot glaze, and top with diced Ruby Red Kraut (page 43).

Coconut Brown Rice Pudding

This recipe makes great use of leftover rice, turning it into a lightly sweet and creamy treat that you can feel great indulging in. Serve warm with a dollop of whipped cream, coconut cream, or maple syrup if you want.

Try adding spices like nutmeg, ginger, cardamom, or cloves if you want to mix it up a bit. Toasted nuts make nice additions as well. It's easy to finish off any leftovers in the morning for breakfast; no one has to know it's not oatmeal.

Put the rice, coconut milk, and almond milk in a medium pot and bring to a simmer over low heat. Cook, stirring frequently, until the mixture thickens a bit and takes on a creamy consistency, 5 to 8 minutes. Stir in the cinnamon, maple syrup, and cherries, and cook until the cherries soften, another 2 to 3 minutes. Remove the pot from the heat and let the pudding cool slightly.

Take the kraut out of the jar with a clean fork, letting any extra brine drain back into it. Finely mince the kraut and stir it into the rice.

Makes 4 to 6 servings

3 cups cooked brown rice (see Rice, page 214, for cooking instructions)

¾ cups canned coconut milk

¾ cups almond milk, or milk of your choice

1 teaspoon ground cinnamon

3 tablespoons maple syrup

⅔ cup dried cherries or raisins, roughly chopped (optional)

½ cup Classic Kraut (page 29)

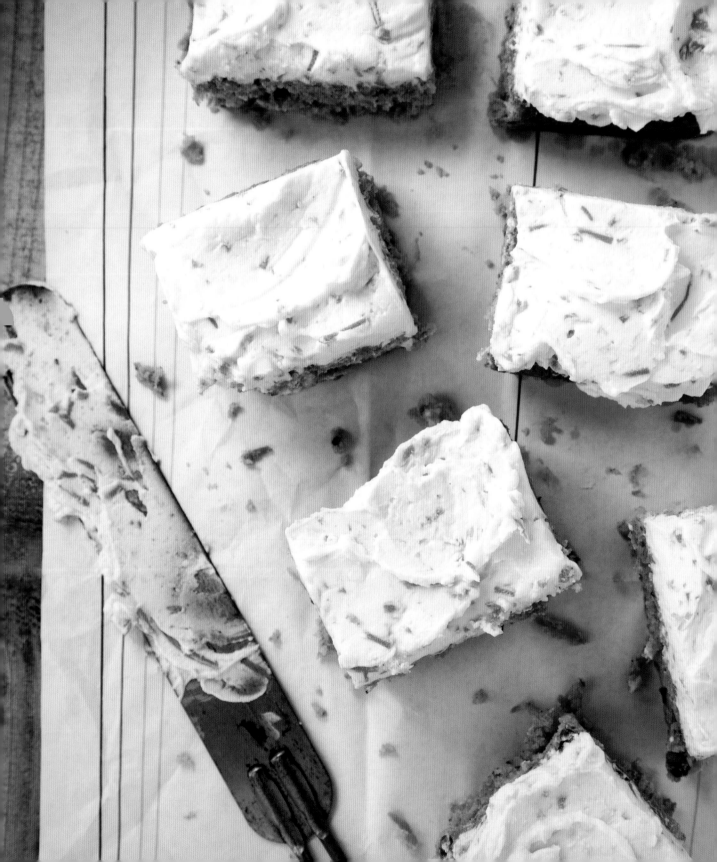

Carrot Bars with Carrot Cream Frosting

The marriage of the familiar flavors of carrot cake and zucchini bread creates these dense, cake-like bars. Firefly's kitchen manager, Linda Harkness, came up with the concept one day when we had heaps of extra Yin Yang Carrots on hand. The first recipe she tried made a very fermented-tasting cake, but we loved the idea and tried several more variations, adding zucchini and fresh carrots to create a lighter and sweeter result.

While we sacrifice a few good microbes in the baking, there are plenty of raw Yin Yang Carrots in the frosting, a zippy, gingery addition to the sweet cream cheese.

These moist and hearty bars make a great healthy dessert or snack and are totally kid- and picky eater–approved. Make them gluten-free by substituting an all-purpose gluten-free baking mix for the flours, and plan on a few extra minutes in the oven.

Preheat the oven to 350 degrees F and thoroughly grease a 9-by-13-inch baking dish.

In a large bowl, whisk together the flours, cinnamon, baking soda, baking powder, nutmeg, and salt.

In another large bowl, using an electric mixer or by hand, beat the melted butter and brown sugar until light and creamy. Add the eggs one at a time, beating until incorporated after each addition. Add the yogurt and beat to combine. Mix the dry ingredients into the butter mixture until well combined.

Take the carrots out of the jar with a clean fork, letting any extra brine drain back into it, and add them to the batter, along with the fresh carrots, zucchini, pineapple, and walnuts. Stir until just combined; do not overmix.

Spread the batter into the prepared baking dish and bake until a knife or toothpick inserted in the center of the pan comes out clean, 35 to 40 minutes.

continued

Makes 16 to 20 bars

- 1½ cups unbleached, all-purpose flour
- ½ cup whole-wheat pastry flour
- 1 teaspoon ground cinnamon
- 1 teaspoon baking soda
- ½ teaspoon baking powder
- ½ teaspoon ground nutmeg
- ½ teaspoon salt
- ¾ cup (1½ sticks) butter or coconut oil, melted
- 1 cup packed brown sugar
- 3 organic eggs
- 1 cup plain or vanilla yogurt
- ½ cup Yin Yang Carrots (page 55)
- 1½ cups (about 2 medium) finely grated carrots

1 medium zucchini (about
    1 cup)

¾ cup crushed canned pineap-
    ple, drained (optional)

¾ cup chopped walnuts
    (optional)

FOR THE FROSTING:

½ cup Yin Yang Carrots
    (page 55)

8 ounces cream cheese

¼ cup (½ stick) butter

1 cup confectioners' sugar

While the cake is baking, make the frosting. Take the carrots out of the jar with a clean fork, letting any extra brine drain back into it. Mince the carrots. In a medium bowl, using an electric mixer or by hand, mix the carrots with the cream cheese, butter, and confectioners' sugar until smooth and creamy.

Put the pan on a rack and let the cake thoroughly cool. When it has cooled, invert the pan over a large plate or platter. Frost the cake, and cut it into squares or rectangles. Serve the bars at room temperature.

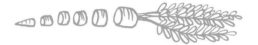

Yin Yang Carrot Balls

You know the feeling. You get home from work and just need something to nibble on. These Yin Yang Carrot Balls are the ultimate fix. They're packed with filling and energizing protein, fiber, healthy fats, and, of course, good-for-your-belly probiotics. Plus, they're only a tad sweet, just enough to satiate your sweet tooth. Pack them for work, a hike, the gym, or while traveling to ensure you always have a healthy snack on hand. They also make a great addition to cheese plates.

Put the chia seeds in a small bowl and add enough water to cover them. Let them soak for at least 15 minutes or up to 1 hour.

Take the carrots out of the jar with a clean fork, letting any extra brine drain back into it. Put them in a colander, let them drain for 10 to 15 minutes, mince them, and set them aside.

Put the dates, ½ cup of the coconut, walnuts, maple syrup, cinnamon, salt, and oats in a food processor. Whirl until the ingredients are evenly broken down, but not quite smooth. Add the chia seeds and carrots, and blend until the ingredients are combined. The mixture will start to clump together like dough—it should be easy to form into a ball with your fingertips. If the mixture is too wet, add oats 1 tablespoon at a time until you get a dough-like consistency.

Put the remaining ¼ cup coconut in a shallow bowl or high-rimmed plate, and have a plate ready for the balls.

Turn the dough out onto a clean work surface. Break off a small piece, and shape it into a 1-inch ball by rolling it between the palms of your hands. Roll the ball in the dried coconut until it's evenly coated, and put it on the plate. Repeat the process with the remaining dough and coconut.

Refrigerate the balls for at least 30 minutes before serving. Serve chilled or at room temperature. To store, refrigerate for up to 5 days or freeze for up to 4 months.

Makes about 2 dozen balls

2 tablespoons chia seeds

1 cup Yin Yang Carrots (page 55)

10 medium dates, pitted

¾ cup unsweetened dried coconut flakes, divided

½ cup walnuts

1 tablespoon maple syrup

1 teaspoon ground cinnamon

Pinch of salt

⅔ cup rolled oats, plus more for thickening if needed

Sweet and Sauer Chocolate Pudding

Traditional chocolate pudding is utterly transformed by the addition of a little Classic Kraut. Once minced, the texture of the kraut disappears into the decadent pudding, but its lively, piquant flavor balances the chocolate's intensity.

Try mixing this with the orange cream filling from the Spiced Roulade (page 197) for a unique orange-accented chocolate cream that you can enjoy on its own or use as a filling for cream puffs, tarts, parfaits, or cakes. Feel free to add more kraut if you like its effervescent flavor.

Makes 2 heaping cups of decadent pudding

½ cup sugar

¾ cup cocoa powder

2 tablespoons cornstarch

¼ teaspoon salt

1½ cups whole milk

½ cup half-and-half or light cream

½ cup semisweet chocolate chips, or 4 ounces bittersweet chocolate, finely chopped

1 teaspoon vanilla extract

⅓ cup Classic Kraut (page 29)

Whisk together the sugar, cocoa powder, cornstarch, and salt in a medium saucepan over low heat. Slowly pour in the milk and half-and-half, whisking constantly until combined. Increase the heat to medium and cook, continuing to stir, until the mixture thickens to the consistency of pudding, 5 to 8 minutes.

Stir in the chocolate chips and cook until the chocolate has melted, 2 to 3 minutes. Stir in the vanilla and cook for another 2 minutes. Remove the pan from the heat and let the pudding cool.

Take the kraut out of the jar with a clean fork, letting any extra brine drain back into it, and finely mince the kraut. Squeeze any excess brine from the kraut. When the pudding has completely cooled, add the minced kraut and stir until well combined. Refrigerate until ready to serve. Serve chilled.

CHOCOLATE IS FERMENTED?!

Before becoming chocolate, cacao beans must first be fermented to rid them of the astringent tannins that make them intensely bitter. Fermenting the beans also darkens their color and enriches their flavor, which is what makes chocolate so decadent.

Acknowledgments

We are so incredibly thankful to our extended Firefly Kitchens family, our volunteers, and our crew for their endless support, encouragement, and hands-on help for the last five years. We thank you and the many others who have supported us in creating this book.

Big thanks to Gary Luke and Susan Roxborough from Sasquatch Books for providing this opportunity to share our love of ferments with a larger audience, and making this book a reality. Christy Cox and Michelle Hope Anderson and the rest of the Sasquatch team, we are most appreciative of all the technical support on this project. Joyce Hwang, Julie Hopper, and Charity Burggraaf, your design, food styling, and photography are brilliant.

Kim O'Donnel and Sally Ekus, thanks for your support and guidance. Ingrid Emerick and Elizabeth Wales, your support and advice about the details of all the unknowns about creating a book were amazing.

Jane Jeszeck and Kitty Harmon, your packaging and presentation of our words, ideas, and recipes into a lovely proposal was what launched this book into being. You have both been so generous and supportive of Firefly since our beginning, and this is proof of that.

Leslie Miller, Kate Rogers, Sandor Katz, Karen Andonian, Adrienne McLaughlin, Rebecca Staffel, and Christi Stapleton, a thousand thanks for your conversations, feedback, and research. Suzanne Cameron, we are forever grateful for all that you do for Firefly Kitchens. Cynthia Lair, thanks for being an inspiration and sharing the love of ferments.

Carol Brown, so many thanks to you for your incredible writing, organizing, and cleaning up of everything we handed over to you. Nora Dummer, thanks for your dedicated time in the kitchen, word wrangling, and your pleasant advice when asked. Sarah Betts, thanks so much for your support from early Firefly days to your thoughtful contribution of ideas, testing, and overall support. Jordan Smith, many thanks for contributing your knowledge and time to our fermentation chapter, recipe testing, and your all-around scientific support of Firefly Kitchens.

The recipe development has been a joy, and wouldn't have been possible without the creative help, counseling, and feedback from so many dear friends. Bebette Cazelais, Betsy Power, Cathy Mowbray, Cathy Sander, Kim O'Donnell, Linda Harkness, Linda Stratton, Michelle Fasser, Mary Ingraham, Teri Adolfo, and Theresa Klaassen, a heartfelt thanks. Also to our recipe testers Amanda, Amber, Andrea, Becky, Beth, Deneen, Carolyn, Cicely, Cindy, Christina, Christine, Colin, Debra, Diane, Elyse, Emily, Erin, Heather, Kandi, Kristen, Ian, Jill, Jocelyn, Josh, Julian, Katie, Linda, Nick, Mathew, Maureen, Melanie, Molly, Rachel, Rebecca, Renee, Sheryl, Taryn, Travis, Tyler, and Virginia (and our apologies for those we missed), we thank you for your time and feedback towards this very important part of the process.

To all the co-ops, independents, and the natural food chains, thank you for believing in fermented foods and buying our products. We also want to thank Whole Foods Market and especially Denise Breyley for promoting our foods throughout their stores. We love and appreciate the work done by the Good Food Awards, for helping to educate the public and celebrate all of us who are making these traditional foods in modern times. And to all the people who have shared their stories of health and healing, of fermented family traditions, and the creative ways that you eat these foods daily . . . each and every one of you have contributed in one way or another to Firefly Kitchens and this cookbook.

From Richard:

This has truly been a journey, beginning the day the call came in from Sasquatch Books, through the development of the many unique and wonderful recipes contained on these pages, to the finale when we proudly held the completed book in our hands.

I want to extend heartfelt thanks to my family, my wife, Jo-Ann, and my daughters, Emily and Charlotte. You have all been unwavering supporters by working in the kitchen, enthusiastically sampling our products at stores and events, and are ongoing ambassadors of the foods we create at Firefly Kitchens. I am so grateful for your support and understanding in light of the demands that have come with starting a business and especially during the writing of this book. Thank you for your commitment and love, and for the grace with which you so freely give both.

From Julie:

Mike, Elliott, and Wyatt O'Brien, what a gift you are to me! While I know you would rather that I made pies or cookies for a living, you have all been so engaged from the start of Firefly and throughout the creation of this book. You guys are simply the best and I appreciate you so incredibly much. Jessa Garibay, thanks for being that loving and positive daughter I never had. Your help in the kitchen and with all these creations will never be forgotten. Ron, Jean, and Janet Bolton, you are the best family anyone could ever ask for and I am so grateful for all the love and nurturing you continuously share. Your constant enthusiasm and belief in Firefly Kitchens and this cookbook means the world to me.

Linnea O'Brien, I love how you have embraced these foods and so willingly share them with others. I appreciate all the testing and collaborating you have done. Diane O'Brien, thanks for your loving support and all the diligent testing. Robyn O'Brien, please continue, "shedding the light on our food system." Your continuous encouragement warms my heart. Julie Hamilton, thanks for being such an inspiration to me, sharing the last thirty-six years of cooking together, and for being a stellar support this last year both in and out of the kitchen. Peggy Lynch, you are an important force in my life. I'm so grateful for all the testing, listening, reading, and feedback you have given me over the years and with this book.

And a huge, heartfelt thanks to all the others who supported me along the way.

Recipes by Kraut

Cooking Rice, Legumes, + Quinoa

In this section, we want to convey the power of planning ahead so you have the ingredients on hand to throw together a healthy meal in minutes. Thinking about your meals ahead of time will help make them easier to prepare and more nutritious.

Spend some time over the weekend or in the early part of the week preparing grains and legumes so you have them handy to use in the recipes that call for them. Or you could invent your own impromptu dish by tossing some greens, legumes, and kraut in a bowl or adding precooked grains or legumes to soups, stews, sides, and stir-fries.

Rice

Although soaking rice isn't necessary, it reduces the cooking time and, more importantly, removes harmful phytates, naturally occurring enzyme inhibitors that make it more difficult for your body to digest the rice and absorb its nutrients.

Cooked rice will keep for 5 to 7 days in the refrigerator.

Type	Amount	Soaking time	Water	Approximate cooking time	Yield
Black	1 cup	2 to 8 hours	1¾ cups	22 to 28 minutes	3 cups
Brown, basmati	1 cup	2 to 8 hours	1¾ cups	18 to 25 minutes	3 cups
Brown, short or long grain	1 cup	8 to 12 hours	1¾ cups	18 to 25 minutes	3 cups

SOAKING. Measure the rice, put it in a large bowl, and add enough water to cover by 2 inches. Let it soak at room temperature for the time indicated in the table above. Thoroughly drain the rice before cooking.

COOKING. Put the soaked rice, a pinch of salt, and fresh water in a medium pot. Bring the water to a boil over medium heat. Lower the heat and simmer until all the liquid is absorbed, or for the indicated cooking time. (Depending on the age and dryness of the rice and how well you drained it, the cooking time will vary.) When the rice is cooked, fluff it with a fork to prevent clumping.

Legumes

As with rice, soaking legumes greatly reduces cooking time and removes harmful phytates.

Cooked legumes will keep for 5 days in the refrigerator.

Type	Amount	Soaking time	Water	Approximate cooking time	Yield
Adzuki beans	2 cups	8 to 12 hours	6 cups	1 to 4 hours	6 cups
Black beans	2 cups	8 to 12 hours	6 cups	1 to 2 hours	6 cups
Chickpeas	2 cups	8 to 12 hours	6 cups	1 to 2 hours	6 cups
Lentils, brown or green	2 cups	None	6 cups	30 minutes to 1 hour	6 cups
Lima beans	2 cups	None	6 cups	1½ hour	6 cups
White beans	2 cups	8 to 12 hours	6 cups	1 to 2 hours	6 cups

SOAKING. Measure the legumes, put them in a large bowl, and add enough water to cover by 2 inches. Let them soak at room temperature for the time indicated in the table above. Drain the legumes before cooking.

COOKING. Put the legumes and fresh water in a large pot. (*Don't* salt the cooking water—the early addition of salt will make your beans tough.) Bring the water to a boil over medium heat. Lower the heat and simmer, testing the legumes occasionally for softness, for the indicated cooking time, or until the legumes are tender and no longer chewy. (Depending on the age and dryness of the legumes, the cooking time will vary. Fresher legumes will cook faster; dryer or older legumes will take a bit longer.) When the legumes are done, drain off any remaining cooking liquid.

Quinoa

Commonly mistaken for a grain, this gluten-free seed—red, white, or multicolored—contains all nine essential amino acids, making it a great plant-based source of complete protein.

Cooked quinoa will keep for 5 days in the refrigerator.

Type	Amount	Rinsing time	Water	Approximate cooking time	Yield
Quinoa	1 cup	1 minute	2 cups	15 to 18 minutes	3 cups

RINSING. Although quinoa doesn't need to be soaked like rice and legumes, it does need to be rinsed to remove the bitter powdery residue that coats each grain. Measure the quinoa, put it in a fine-mesh strainer, and rinse it thoroughly under cold water for at least 30 seconds. Thoroughly drain the quinoa before cooking.

COOKING. Put fresh water in a medium pot. Bring the water to a boil over high heat. Add the rinsed quinoa and a pinch of salt, reduce the heat to low, cover the pot, and simmer for the indicated cooking time, or until all the water has been absorbed. Remove the pan from the heat, and gently fluff the quinoa with a fork.

Not-So-Common Ingredients

CHIA SEEDS. A member of the sage family, these seeds are incredibly high in protein and fiber, while relatively mild in taste. When soaked, they absorb a great amount of liquid and create a mucilaginous gel that's great on its own as a pudding or mixed into smoothies or baked goods.

COCONUT OIL. Coconut oil, which is solid at room temperature, can be heated to higher temperatures than other oils before oxidizing. This means that you can use coconut oil to sear, sauté, and bake without consuming oxidized fat, which has been linked to many health issues, including cancer growth and high cholesterol. Coconut oil is also a potent antibacterial and contains a type of saturated fat called lauric acid, which has been shown to increase "good" HDL cholesterol. It imparts a delicious, mellow, nutty sweetness to foods.

FARRO. This nutty and slightly chewy whole grain is very versatile and comes in several different varieties.

FISH SAUCE *(Nam pla* or *nuoc mam).* Made from fermented fish, this Southeast Asian staple is very pungent, salty, and complex. The unique flavor that fish sauce provides is not an easy one to replicate.

GHEE. Typically used in Indian cuisine, ghee is clarified butter, which is prepared by simmering the butter to remove the milk solids and water. Ghee is said to stimulate the secretion of stomach acids to help with digestion. Ghee is shelf-stable and doesn't require refrigeration.

HEMP SEEDS. High in omega-3 and omega-6 fatty acids, hemp seeds are considered to be one of the most nutrient-dense foods on the planet. They're deliciously nutty in flavor and creamy in texture.

KEFIR. Another food rich in probiotics, kefir is a fermented dairy product that contains an abundance of vitamins, minerals, and essential amino acids. Slightly sour and carbonated, it's often thought of as drinkable yogurt. Though traditionally made from raw cow's milk, kefir is also produced from coconut milk and coconut water.

KOREAN RED PEPPER *(gochugaru).* Slighty smoky and sweet, this traditional pepper come in a finely ground powder or flakes and is best without the addition of salt or other additives.

MILLET. Gluten-free and subtly flavored, this seed makes a great substitution for many common cooking grains.

MISO. Miso is a traditional food from Japan made from fermented soy beans, barley, or rice. It's high in protein, vitamins, and minerals.

NORI. Very thin sheets of dried seaweed typically used for rolling sushi. *Yakinori* is toasted nori and all varieties are high in protein, vitamins, calcium and iron.

QUINOA. Complete with all eight essential amino acids, this seed is a complete protein and when cooked it will expand to about 4 times its original size. Mild in flavor, it easily accepts most seasonings.

RICE VERMICELLI NOODLES. Sometimes referred to as rice noodles or rice sticks, these are gluten-free noodles made from rice flour and water. They're traditionally used in Southeast Asian dishes, such as soups, salads, or stir-fries.

SMOKED PAPRIKA (*pimentón*). This sweet and smoky paprika, a newly popular spice, is made from dried pimento peppers that have been smoked over a fire and ground into a fine powder.

TAHINI. Sesame seeds are hulled and ground to create this creamy and thick condiment, commonly used in Turkish and Middle Eastern cuisine. Tahini is an essential ingredient in hummus, baba ghanoush, and halvah, a confection of sesame seeds and honey.

TRUFFLE OIL OR TRUFFLE SALT. Truffles, with their robust flavor and pungent aroma, are arguably the most sought-after mushrooms in the world. Because of their high price and rarity on the market, their essence is added to oil and salt to easily enhance the flavor of dishes.

WASABI POWDER OR PASTE. Wasabi is oftentimes referred to as Japanese horseradish, despite its being an entirely different plant. This strong and spicy root is commonly used as a condiment.

Sources for Specialty Ingredients

- Amazon.com

Amazon sells almost any food item or kitchen gadget you can imagine, including chia seeds, hemp seeds, and wasabi powder and Korean Red Pepper.

- BobsRedMill.com

Based out of Oregon, Bob's Red Mill grows practically any whole grain you can think of (and many that you may never have heard of), including millet, polenta, and farro.

- CBsNuts.com

CB's is our go-to peanut butter. We appreciate the company's commitment to nuts and seeds grown in the United States, and its dedication to the freshness guaranteed by small-batch roasting.

- CelticSeaSalt.com

Since 1976, Celtic Sea Salt has produced its unprocessed and mineral-rich sea salt, Firefly Kitchens' salt of choice.

- DavidsonCommodities.com/pnw-coop-specialty-foods

We love the variety of heirloom lentils and special chickpeas from this Pacific Northwest Farmers Cooperative. Dedicated to preserving family farms and using traditional growing practices, it sells only GMO-free products.

- MatizEspana.com

Matiz España imports high-quality ingredients from various regions in Spain—including smoked paprika (pimentón), sea salt, olive oils, and vinegars.

- Nutiva.com

Nutiva is a solid source for organic hemp foods, coconut oil, and chia seeds, and donates 1 percent of all sales to sustainable agriculture groups.

Our Favorite Books

Gut and Psychology Syndrome by Natasha Campbell-McBride, MD (Medinform Publishing, 2010)

> A pioneer of probiotics, Natasha Campbell-McBride makes a compelling argument for the link between poor digestive health and many ailments of the mind and body. Attributing learning disabilities in children, from autism and ADHD to dyslexia and depression, to a lack of beneficial bacteria, Campbell-McBride presents groundbreaking research and recommendations for how to improve both physical and mental health for children and people of any age.

Nourishing Traditions by Sally Fallon (New Trends Publishing, 2003)

> Hugely influential and at times slightly controversial, *Nourishing Traditions* is a cornerstone for many modern nutritionists. This was the book that hooked us both on fermentation and has since become a big part of our food philosophy. We continue to return to it for its wealth of information, stories, and traditional recipes.

Mastering Fermentation by Mary Karlin (Ten Speed Press, 2013)

> Featuring more than seventy recipes, *Mastering Fermentation* includes everything from making simple mustards and vinegars to fermenting meat and curing fish. With a detailed glossary and a resource list, this visually stunning book is a great reference for anyone interested in fermentation.

Wild Fermentation by Sandor Ellix Katz (Chelsea Green Publishing, 2003)

> This is one of the earliest books published on fermentation. It will be an inspiration to the novice fermenter and remains a fine book on how to ferment many foods.

The Art of Fermentation by Sandor Ellix Katz (Chelsea Green Publishing, 2012)
> Often referred to as the bible of fermentation, *The Art of Fermentation* presents a deep and thoroughly researched look at the concepts and processes of food preservation. For both the novice and the professional, this book is a profound work for understanding and practicing fermentation.

Making Sauerkraut and Pickled Vegetables at Home by Klaus Kaufmann and Annelies Schöneck (Books Alive, 1997)
> We love this book and often give it out when we teach classes at Firefly Kitchens. It's concise yet thorough, and is packed with fermentation facts, recipes, and descriptions of many of the health benefits of fermented foods.

Digestive Wellness by Elizabeth Lipski (McGraw-Hill, 2011)
> This is a great resource for anyone suffering from digestive discomfort or wanting to eat fermented foods on their journey to better health. Lipski goes into great detail about many common conditions and discusses what you can do to take your health into your own hands.

The World Healthiest Foods by George Mateljan (George Mateljan Foundation, 2007)
> This book features nutrient content, best preparation methods, and simple, tasty recipes for hundreds of veggies, fruits, and grains. If you're interested in what nutrients your foods contain and how to best prepare them to preserve those benefits, this is the book for you.

Full Moon Feast by Jessica Prentice (Chelsea Green Publishing, 2006)
> Prentice is one of the owners of Three Stone Hearth, where we both apprenticed, and where the idea for Firefly Kitchens was first hatched. Exploring food culturally and seasonally, she takes a traditional approach to meal preparation, insisting we reconnect with our food system. This book is a great reminder to appreciate food in its simplest and purest form, and has some wonderful and approachable recipes.

Fermented Foods for Health by Deirdre Rawlings, PhD, ND (Fair Winds Press, 2013)
> In this wonderful little book, Rawlings goes into some depth about the science behind fermentation and the effects of bacteria on the digestive and immune systems, offers detailed advice about how fermented foods can strengthen immunity and prevent illness, and provides recipes.

Index

Note: Photographs are indicated by *italics*.

Conversions

VOLUME

UNITED STATES	METRIC	IMPERIAL
¼ tsp.	1.25 ml	
½ tsp.	2.5 ml	
1 tsp.	5 ml	
½ Tbsp.	7.5 ml	
1 Tbsp.	15 ml	
⅛ c.	30 ml	1 fl. oz.
¼ c.	60 ml	2 fl. oz.
⅓ c.	80 ml	2.5 fl. oz.
½ c.	125 ml	4 fl. oz.
1 c.	250 ml	8 fl. oz.
2 c. (1 pt.)	500 ml	16 fl. oz.
1 qt.	1 l	32 fl. oz.

LENGTH

UNITED STATES	METRIC
⅛ in.	3 mm
¼ in.	6 mm
½ in.	1.25 cm
1 in.	2.5 cm
1 ft.	30 cm

WEIGHT

AVOIRDUPOIS	METRIC
¼ oz.	7 g
½ oz.	15 g
1 oz.	30 g
2 oz.	60 g
3 oz.	90 g
4 oz.	115 g
5 oz.	150 g
6 oz.	175 g
7 oz.	200 g
8 oz. (½ lb.)	225 g
9 oz.	250 g
10 oz.	300 g
11 oz.	325 g
12 oz.	350 g
13 oz.	375 g
14 oz.	400 g
15 oz.	425 g
16 oz. (1 lb.)	450 g
1½ lb.	750 g
2 lb.	900 g
2¼ lb.	1 kg
3 lb.	1.4 kg
4 lb.	1.8 kg

TEMPERATURE

OVEN MARK	FAHRENHEIT	CELSIUS	GAS
Very cool	250–275	130–140	½–1
Cool	300	150	2
Warm	325	165	3
Moderate	350	175	4
Moderately hot	375	190	5
	400	200	6
Hot	425	220	7
	450	230	8
Very Hot	475	245	9